STRATEGIC INTERVENTIONS IN MENTAL HEALTH RHETORIC

Offering rhetorically informed strategic interventions, this innovative collection moves beyond critiques of mental health issues, problems, and care. With sections that focus on methodological, cultural and legal, and pedagogical interventions, readers will find an engaging discussion of a discrete mental health phenomenon as well as a clear interventional takeaway in each chapter.

Contributors make use of critical discourse analyses, ethnographic inquiries, autoethnographic inquiries, case studies, and textual analyses to engage such mental health research topics as postpartum depression among Chinese mothers; insanity pleas; anosognosia; issues of intimacy, access, and embodiment in research projects; community support groups; Black mental health; women in Alcoholics Anonymous; and mental health in faculty workshops and university online health tools. The authors and editors create scholarship on mental health that explicitly builds productive methodological, theoretical, and practical bridges among scholars and teachers in the various specialties of writing and communication.

This collection will interest scholars, students, and practitioners in health and medical humanities; rhetoric of health and medicine; health communication; medical anthropology; scientific and technical communication; disability studies; and rhetorical studies generally.

Lisa Melonçon is Professor of Technical Communication at the University of South Florida. She specializes in rhetoric of health and medicine and disability studies.

Cathryn Molloy is Associate Professor and Director of Undergraduate Studies in James Madison University's School of Writing, Rhetoric and Technical Communication.

STRATEGIC INTERVENTIONS IN MENTAL HEALTH RHETORIC

Edited by
Lisa Melonçon and
Cathryn Molloy

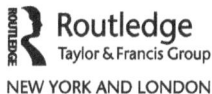

Routledge
Taylor & Francis Group

NEW YORK AND LONDON

Cover art: untitled phone art by Michael Verde

First published 2022
by Routledge
605 Third Avenue, New York, NY 10158

and by Routledge
4 Park Square, Milton Park, Abingdon, Oxon, OX14 4RN

Routledge is an imprint of the Taylor & Francis Group, an informa business

Library of Congress Cataloging-in-Publication Data
Names: Meloncon, Lisa K., editor. | Molloy, Cathryn, editor.
Title: Strategic interventions in mental health rhetoric /
edited by Lisa Melonçon and Cathryn Molloy.
Description: New York, NY : Routledge, 2022. |
Includes bibliographical references and index. |
Identifiers: LCCN 2021040340 (print) |
LCCN 2021040341 (ebook) | ISBN 9780367701581 (hardback) |
ISBN 9780367697600 (paperback) | ISBN 9781003144854 (ebook)
Subjects: MESH: Psychosocial Intervention | Sociological Factors |
Mental Health
Classification: LCC RA790.5 (print) | LCC RA790.5 (ebook) |
NLM WM 420.5.P4 | DDC 362.2—dc23
LC record available at https://lccn.loc.gov/2021040340
LC ebook record available at https://lccn.loc.gov/2021040341

ISBN: 9780367701581 (hbk)
ISBN: 9780367697600 (pbk)
ISBN: 9781003144854 (ebk)

DOI: 10.4324/9781003144854

Typeset in Bembo
by codeMantra

CONTENTS

FIGURES

TABLES

ACKNOWLEDGMENTS

We put out the call for papers for this collection just as COVID-19 cases began to be widely reported in China; by the time we notified authors of their acceptance and asked them to prepare full first drafts of their chapters, many were facing a wide variety of challenges associated with the pandemic. Still, they brought exceptional energy, creativity, thoughtfulness, and intellectual rigor to their work. We, therefore, want to acknowledge them and their extraordinary efforts during particularly daunting times first and foremost.

This work grew out of the extremely generous community of rhetoric of health and medicine scholars, and we thank this community for inspiring and supporting the work in this collection.

We also thank our coeditor at the *Rhetoric of Health and Medicine* journal J. Blake Scott and our mutual mentor J. Fred Reynolds for their constant encouragement and support as we worked through this project.

Lisa would like to thank the University of South Florida's College of Arts and Sciences and the Department of English for their support, and Cathryn, likewise, thanks her colleagues in James Madison University's School of Writing, Rhetoric and Technical Communication.

We would both like to extend our enormous gratitude to Ms. Jessie Wiggins for her sharp and generous copy edits and Haley Jones for her assistance with the index. We both also want to thank Michael Verde for his enormous generosity in giving us permission to use his phone art piece for the cover of the book. Merci beaucoup.

Finally, last, but certainly not least, a big "thank-you" goes to our families for all of their love and support.

CONTRIBUTORS

Editors

Lisa Melonçon is Professor of Technical Communication at the University of South Florida. Dr. Melonçon specializes in rhetoric of health and medicine and disability studies. She is coeditor of *Rhetoric of Health and Medicine As/Is* (2020); *Methodologies for the Rhetoric of Health and Medicine* (2018); and editor of *Rhetorical Accessibility: At the Intersection of Technical Communication and Disability Studies* (2013).

Cathryn Molloy is Associate Professor and Director of Undergraduate Studies in James Madison University's School of Writing, Rhetoric and Technical Communication. Her work has appeared in *Rhetoric Society Quarterly, Qualitative Inquiry, College English, Technical Communication Quarterly,* and *Rhetoric Review.* She is the author of *Rhetorical Ethos in Health and Medicine: Patient Credibility, Stigma, and Misdiagnosis* and coeditor of the volume *Women's Health Advocacy Rhetorical Ingenuity for the 21st Century.*

Contributors

Leslie R. Anglesey is Assistant Professor in the Department of English at Sam Houston State University. Her research focuses on accessible health communication and accessible writing pedagogy. Her work has appeared in *The Peer Review, Prompt: A Journal of Academic Writing Assignments*, and *Works and Days.* Her coedited collection, *Standing at the Threshold: Working Through Liminality in the Composition and Rhetoric TAship*, is forthcoming from Utah State University Press. Additional information about her research and teaching is available at: leslieanglesey.com.

Lora Arduser is Associate Professor in Technical and Professional Writing at the University of Cincinnati. Her research is situated in the rhetoric of health and medicine and focuses on rhetorics of expertise and rhetoric, gender, and technology. She is author of *Living Chronic: Agency and Expertise in the Rhetoric of Diabetes* (2017). Her research has also been published in *Technical Communication Quarterly, Journal of Technical Writing and Communication, Women's Studies in Communication, Computers and Composition*, and *Narrative Inquiry*.

Nora Augustine holds a Ph.D. in English with a Graduate Certificate in Women's and Gender Studies from the University of North Carolina at Chapel Hill. Her research and advocacy work center on mental health, social justice, and the rhetorical functions of auto/biographical writing. For her contributions to the Chapel Hill community, she has received a Maynard Adams Fellowship for the Public Humanities and a Senior Fellowship through the UNC Humanities Professional Pathway program.

Rachael Blasiman is Associate Professor in the Department of Psychological Sciences at Kent State University at Salem. She completed her Ph.D. in Experimental Psychology at Case Western Reserve University and teaches psychology courses, mentors student researchers, and engages in research on student success.

Tianna Cobb is Postdoctoral Fellow in the Department of Communication at George Mason University where she focuses on Health and Organizational Communication. Her research examines the normalization of mental wellness within the Black community. As an applied communication scholar, her research and teaching are situated in health activism at the praxis of dismantling systems of oppression, exposing health inequities, and highlighting marginalized voices and experiences.

Lisa DeTora is Associate Professor and the Director of STEM Writing at Hofstra University. Her interests in medical humanities and embodiment seminars have led to book chapters on domestic violence rhetoric and intersex embodiments as well as two coedited volumes, *Bodies in Transition in the Health Humanities* (Routledge 2020) and *Graphic Embodiments* (Leuven 2021). Additional scholarship has appeared in RHM, CDQ, JTWC, and various medical journals.

Barbara George is Assistant Professor in English at the Kent Salem campus. She received a Ph.D. in English from Kent State University. Barbara has researched student retention efforts as related to literacies and also researches language and environmental justice.

Mark A. Hannah is Associate Professor of English at Arizona State University. His scholarship examines the intersections of law, rhetoric, and expertise in multidisciplinary problem-solving contexts. His work has appeared in a range of edited collections and journals including *Nevada Law Journal, IEEE: Transactions on Professional Communication, Technical Communication, Technical Communication Quarterly, Journal of Technical Writing and Communication, Communication Design Quarterly, Connexions International Professional Communication Journal, College Composition and Communication, Nature,* and others.

Adam Hubrig is Assistant Professor in the Department of English at Sam Houston State University. Their research centers on disability and neurodivergence in composition and writing studies, community literacy, queer rhetoric, and English education. Their work has appeared in *Pedagogy, Community Literacy Journal, College Composition and Communication,* and *The Journal of Multimodal Rhetorics.* They reside in Huntsville, TX, with their partner and cats.

Lori J. Joseph is Associate Professor of Communication Studies, Affiliate Professor of Gender and Women's Studies, and the Director of Public Health at Hollins University in Roanoke, VA. Joseph's research and teaching interests include women's work narratives, gender and work, and gender and health. Working with a student team, she recently completed the project, "Proceeding" that focuses on Ann Hopkins, a Hollins University alumnae who won a Supreme Court decision against Price Waterhouse for gender discrimination in the workplace.

Sean Kamperman is Assistant Professor of English at Valparaiso University. Kamperman's research examines rhetorical issues such as ethos, credibility, and communicative competence in relation to community literacy and disability rights. His work has appeared in the *Gayle Morris Sweetland Digital Rhetoric Collaborative, Disability Studies Quarterly,* and *Critical Education.*

Stephanie Kelley-Romano is Associate Professor and Chair of Rhetoric, Film, and Screen Studies at Bates College in Lewiston, Maine. Her research and teaching interests include gender and media, myth and narrative, conspiracy, political rhetoric, and the public sphere. Her research has appeared in such venues as *Newsweek, The Journal of Hate Studies, Communication Quarterly, Journalism Studies,* and *The Journal of UFO Studies.*

Lynn Reid is Assistant Professor of Rhetoric and Composition and Director of Basic Writing at Fairleigh Dickinson University. Dr. Reid's research interests include basic writing, digital literacies and multimodal composition, and writing program administration. Her work has appeared in *WPA Journal*, *Journal of Basic Writing*, *TESOL Encyclopedia*, and several edited collections. Dr. Reid is a current cochair of the Council on Basic Writing, a CCCC standing group and serves as Associate Editor for the *Basic Writing e-Journal*.

Tomeka Robinson is Senior Associate Dean of the Honors College & Professor of Rhetoric & Public Advocacy at Hofstra University. Dr. Robinson's scholarly interests lie at the intersections of health, culture, and policy. Dr. Robinson is also very active within several professional and civic organizations including the Long Island Community and Academic Research Partnership, Pi Kappa Delta National Forensics Honorary Association, and the International Forensics Association.

Cynthia Ryan is Associate Professor of English at the University of Alabama at Birmingham, where she teaches courses in science writing, medical writing, and magazine writing. Coeditor of *The Rhetoric of Health and Medicine As/Is: Theories and Approaches for the Field* (2020) and Associate Editor of *RHM Journal*, Cynthia has written for the *LA Times*, *Chicago Tribune*, *Cancer Today*, and *Salon. com*. She also founded Street Smarts™, a cancer education program for homeless women in Birmingham, AL.

Susie Salmon is Director of Legal Writing and Clinical Professor of Law at the University of Arizona, James E. Rogers College of Law. Her scholarship explores how long-standing practices and values in legal education affect access to justice, bias in the profession, lawyer/law student well-being, and the legal profession. She is coauthor of *The Moot Court Advisors Handbook*, and her work has appeared in a range of law reviews including *Legal Communication & Rhetoric: JAWLD*.

Hua Wang, Senior Lecturer in the College of Engineering at Cornell University, is a scholar whose research focuses on the rhetoric of health and medicine with a focus on technical communication, particularly in the Chinese context. Her dissertation examines the expression of rhetorical agency in a childbirth and pregnancy commercial app in China; she maps the extent to which the app spreads empowering information about pregnancy and mothering to its users (Chinese women). Her work has appeared in the *Journal of Technical Writing and Communication* and *Technical Communication Quarterly*.

INTRODUCTION

Interventions in Mental Health Rhetoric Research

Cathryn Molloy and Lisa Melonçon

As we compose this introductory chapter, we're in the thick of an ongoing global pandemic that is unfolding alongside protests calling for long awaited racial justice. These national and international events usher in a host of new mental health concerns, or possibly reignite preexisting mental health problems. Indeed, experts warn that a mental health pandemic is developing alongside the COVID-19 pandemic—that long after restrictions lift and cases and deaths decline, the mental health ramifications of this pandemic will persist (Kar et al., 2020; Kumar & Nayar, 2020; Mahase, 2020; Ornell et al., 2020; Pereira-Sanchez et al., 2020). Likewise, those fighting for racial justice face a constant onslaught of traumas; they must live in a constant state of fraught agitation as they quite literally fight for their lives (Gorski, 2019; McKnight-Eily et al., 2021; Nadal et al., 2014).

Even while we share others' alarm at increasing mental health needs, we also acknowledge that, arguably, every moment in human history is rife with the possibility of claiming the existence of new, increased, or accelerated mental health distresses. Likewise, from an academic standpoint, scholarship in mental health rhetoric research (MHRR) is not an overnight concern. In fact, MHRR studies set out to show that mental health problems or mental "illnesses" are mechanisms of social control that reveal more about ideological allegiances than they do about anything approximating "health" per say.

If mental illness labels as oppressive and normative are a frequent refrain, a common topic or *topos* through which this claim is made is via rhetorical examinations of diagnostic practices and tools, such as the proliferation of mental disease categories that are discernable in the succession of editions of the *Diagnostic and Statistical Manual of Mental Disorders* (*DSM*)—currently in its 5th version (Reynolds, 2018). Likewise, if calling attention to suspect diagnostic

DOI: 10.4324/9781003144854-1

and treatment practices using the tools and terms available via rhetoric has been one tact in this body of work (see, e.g., Emmons, 2010; Hanganu-Bresch & Berkenkotter, 2019; McCarthy & Gerring, 1994; Reynolds, 2018), focusing on patient and practitioner experiences with the aim of improving working lives and patient care from rhetorical frameworks has also been a trend (Holladay, 2017; Prendergast, 2001; Price, 2011; Rothfelder & Thornton, 2017; Uthappa, 2017).

What the critical scholarship does quite well, then, is it adds to other efforts in the social sciences and humanities to sound the alarm when questionable claims of mental health "risk" or mental illness "realities" lead to loss of rights and related abuses; likewise, it uses the voices and experiences of those described as "patients" to demonstrate novel uses of language and persuasion meant to push back against overly prescriptive, ableist, stigmatized, or medicalized characterizations (see, e.g., Yergeau & Huebner, 2017). We see this as important work at all times and in all situations.

We contend that the vast world of mental health constitutes a messy object—an object so complex that it eludes researchers' comprehensive assessment (Law, 2004). The very idea of mental health is only surpassed in dubiousness by the idea of a mental illness. Yet, where does this leave those with real day-to-day struggles with mental well-being, as evidenced by a range of ontologies, from nagging feelings of anxiety or paranoia to full-blown panic attacks and delusions? Rather than merely critiquing biomedical approaches to mental health, rather than devaluing biosocial or biopsychosocial approaches, this collection steps into the messy assemblages that constitute day-to-day life with and in mental health concerns by offering concrete things—these interventions—that can be done.

Interventional Rhetoric[1]

In conceptualizing this project, we were drawn to the idea of interventions. The word "interventions," of course, implies an "intermediary" who is "'stepping in', or interfering in any affair, so as to affect its course or issue" (Intervention). The root—intervene—is an action-oriented word that affords a hope for a different result through a direct movement to prevent or to alter an outcome. To intervene invokes a deliberate attempt at change. Interventions in health and medicine, of course, are most widely associated with "public health interventions," which are campaigns or policy approaches designed to improve physical and mental health at the population level. Some well-known examples of such interventions are vaccine campaigns or behavior modifications programs, such as those designed to promote smoking cessation or healthy eating. Public health interventions are also closely associated with evaluation processes meant to determine their effectiveness and to provide information for accountability.

Of course, choosing the word "intervention" in a health and medical context, rhetorical or otherwise, calls up associations of "medical interventions," and social constructivist critiques in the humanities and social sciences point to the dangers of overinterventions into health and medical realities that would be, ironically, better off left alone. These forms of interventions in other fields and disciplines often lack an attention to both the construction and analysis of the communication used, which again highlights the need for a rhetorical approach. For example, the rhetoric of health and medicine literature encompasses work in the rhetorics of reproduction—a body of work that has shown the issues and problems that arise when a natural process like birth is medicalized, leading to iatrogenic consequences (see, e.g., Hensley-Owens, 2015). This example demonstrates the necessity for rhetorical interventions, even as we acknowledge the potential slippage of the term.

But by embracing "interventions" for its forcefulness in making space for MHRR, then, we'd like to push intervention one step further. We want to highlight the necessity of intervention's ability to catalyze *real and specific change* and its propensity to *break down disciplinary silos* in the process. In fact, working across disciplinary divides and engaging in transdisciplinary inquiries, we argue, is necessary for MHRR to continue to move forward. The spirit of this collection is to offer up strategic interventions into MHRR that are immediately useful and usable in multiple disciplines and contexts. The collection does this through a form of theory-building.

Theory Building

Positing "interventions" in conjunction with mental health puts forth a theory-building concept that calls to mind the early work of MHRR and the rhetoric of health and medicine. The latter found its own place within academic and research locations because it became more apparent that the language and communication practices associated with health and medicine needed to be critically analyzed and better understood. Invoking "intervention" as part of his article's title, for example, John Lyne argued that

> To think rhetorically is to reflect constructively on the habits of representation that position people for making judgments. Rhetoric is concerned with the invention of language that enables action, but also with the capacities of language to address and persuade.
>
> *(Lyne, 2001, p. 13)*

Lyne concisely described one of the driving tenets of why rhetoric does indeed matter to health and medicine—that it is through language and rhetoric that biomedicine comes into being and more so, how it can be changed.

We take theory to mean a set of principles on which a practice can be based. This interpretation of theory as something more applied aligns with the past history of MHRR, which has often moved between theory and practice.

Mats Alvesson and Dan Kärreman (2011) suggested that "theory is likely to emerge through the challenging of established patterns rather than through attempts to put the bits of the jigsaw back together" (p. 21), and this conception of theory that pushes back against established boundaries is crucial in broadening the rhetorical understanding of mental health research. Unlike current practices where scholars draw on multiple theories in other disciplines and put them together as an interpretive framework, Alvesson and Kärreman (2011) encouraged active engagement and skepticism with the status quo, and we engage theory similarly. In other words, we propose to do theory-building work because "without an inventive approach to theory, we lose our ability to notice different things in familiar phenomena and sites, and to make sense of happenings in less familiar sites" (Scott & Melonçon, 2018, p. 12). Focusing on intervention, thus, is a deliberate move to work through the question: How can MHRR understand its role within rhetoric, rhetoric of health and medicine, and other related fields and disciplines?

In so doing, we hope this collection shows how MHRR can and should make explicit moves to intervene across disciplines and practices such that the work avoids the pitfall of being merely descriptive of issues and problems in mental health work and/or only admiring of novel linguistic and symbolic forms and becomes, instead, highly impactful and useful across many related areas of study. What has never been given enough attention, is what rhetorical inquiries into mental health might *specifically do* or *should specifically do* out there in the world beyond what we see it doing quite well at present:

- presenting critical accounts of issues and problems inherent in how mental health conditions are diagnosed and how mental healthcare gets done and
- sharing admirable rhetorical moves made by those unfairly characterized as unable to mobilize their own agency.

While engaging with related literature and adding to the vibrant academic bodies of work to which MHRR contributes, the chapters in this book also explicitly focus on *something specific that can be done*, whether it's, for example:

- A newly coined term or concept that **can be put to generative methodological uses** as in Lisa Melonçon and Lora Arduser's introduction of the new term "collective intimacy";
- An activist legal tactic that **can be adapted** to related campaigns as in Mark Hannah and Susie Salmon's recommendations for how to act as a strategic intermediary against stigma; or

- A pedagogical tact against discrimination that **can be taken up** as in Lynn Reid's description of an empathy-driven faculty workshop she developed to dispel misunderstandings of students' mental health.

In keeping with the complex ontologies of mental health conceived broadly, strategic interventions are not as much revelatory as they are necessary. They have utility. They signify the pedestrian and mundane, the just-in-time and because there were no other viable alternatives. Chapters address domains that scholar-activist-practitioners in a variety of interrelated fields of study find themselves working within: research, activism, and teaching/administration.

Preview of Chapters

Interventions put forward in each chapter grow out of rhetorical theories, and thus, use an expansive view of rhetoric to purposefully craft such involvements. Rhetorical interventions are firmly transgressive and, therefore, require tenacity, creativity, and boldness. The chapters in this collection are written with these guiding principles.

Following our own call to consider interventions, this volume constructs the following categories of intervention and is arranged accordingly:

- *methodological interventions* for studying and researching specific communities with approaches aimed at helping future researchers to collect, analyze, and theorize compelling data related to mental health
- *legal, cultural, and institutional interventions* to end stigma and impact material conditions related to specific cultures, laws, and institutions
- *pedagogical and cocurricular interventions* for work with academic programs, student groups, and learning centers—especially as such interventions relate to dispelling misconceptions and promoting the affordances of "mad" subjectivities and/or neurodiversities.

In each section of this book, readers will find chapters that employ a wide variety of methodological approaches (critical discourse analyses, ethnographic inquiries, autoethnographic inquiries, case studies, textual analyses, notable methodological experiments, and hybrid empirical work that folds in autoethnographic data with more traditional forms) to engage such topics as postpartum depression among Chinese mothers; insanity pleas; anosognosia; issues of intimacy, access, and embodiment in research projects; community support groups; women in alcoholics anonymous; faculty workshops; and university online health tools. Recognizing that many fields of study could benefit from this work, the chapters deliver useful content for a wide readership. Rhetoricians, we recognize, are not the only scholars who've shown interest in what a language-based inquiry into the world that mental health inhabits might reveal. This collection is as much for them as it is for scholars in our own diverse field. As mental health concerns are more and more a part of discussions of day-to-day life in academe, too, this collection is also meant for those working in higher education in general.

Brief Chapter Summaries

Following the introductory chapter, readers will find three chapters that offer up methodological interventions. In the first of these chapters, Lisa Melonçon and Lora Arduser's articulation of collective intimacy—a theory that becomes the basis for rethinking the relationship between humans, technology, and information as experienced in online health forums with specific attention to how intimacy is formed. Offering up a term that clarifies the role and importance of patient-to-patient information exchange and using a broad corpus of disparate forums across disease categories, distributed intimacy will be useful to a variety of others attempting to build new theories in a wide variety of research projects. Importantly, Melonçon and Arduser show the payoff of looking across disease categories and online platforms rather than relying on singular sites. Their chapter is, thus, a model for other projects and an intervention into how online health forums are studied; it also puts forward an infinitely useful new term in "collective intimacy."

Sean Kamperman also provides a useful new term in theorizing "inclusive tactics"—a term that formalizes the ways that methodological judgments precipitate from researchers' prior experiences and dispositions. Relying on the case of his own field-based study in rhetoric at a mental health nonprofit, Kamperman describes his own approach to inclusion as emphasizing privacy, autonomy, and self-determination—attributes that helped his research project along in some ways and thwarted its success in others. As a way of productively intervening in future research projects, Kamperman ends his chapter with a useful reflective tool designed to allow researchers to assess the affordances and limitations of their own inclusive tactics. Also offering future researchers a concrete tool, Lisa DeTora and Tomeka Robinson propose a heuristic and narrative framework for developing and refining rhetorical interventions into mental health based on an intersectional, culture-centered approach to communication and domestic violence.

Next, readers will find four chapters focused on legal, cultural, and institutional interventions that are very often activist in nature. Nora Augustine's chapter begins the section by combining textual analysis of support group documentation (curricula, handouts, and facilitator training materials) with autoethnographic inquiry to examine the rhetoric of support groups from the perspective of a facilitator to argue that what she calls the "para-therapeutic rhetoric" of support groups serves an essential function in clarifying participants' past and present relationships to mental health. Ultimately, Augustine's chapter argues, nontraditional care settings like support groups present an unexpected opportunity for MHRR scholar-citizens to be "useful" to their communities by facilitating expressions of uncategorized, but nonetheless transformative, distress.

Stephanie Kelley-Romano and Lori Joseph, then, depict the ways that women make sense of their lived experience in getting, and staying, sober within Alcoholics Anonymous. In articulating these interpretive justifications, the chapter intervenes by giving voice to women's lived experience and identifying sites of tension between expectations of respectability and the authenticity of self. Presenting an analysis that identifies the rhetorical strategies (including redefinition, humor, and transcendence) instrumental to constructing a coherent narrative of recovery for women which remains confined within the bounds of "respectable," the chapter is useful in its articulation of participants' ways of working within and against an established institution to get what they need to get out of the process while not entirely giving themselves over to the language and rhetorics of that institution.

Next, in her culturally responsive chapter, Hua Wang takes up stigma surrounding postpartum depression in China where the condition is often erroneously believed to be the result of new mom's weakness or her negative feelings. As a result, postpartum depression is often misdiagnosed and thus not treated properly. Since postpartum depression ranks second among China's top mental problems, and Chinese public awareness of postpartum depression is very low, many women do not seek psychological help, avoid medical treatment, and receive little support from their families for their postpartum depression. In some cases, the condition is an aggravating factor of self-harm and suicide. Analyzing how women knitters actively participate in shaping crucial spaces for identification in online and real-life spaces, Wang offers a model of community care when conditions do not easily allow for the possibility of other forms of care. Wang's chapter, thus, offers a model of culturally specific, community-based, and online antistigma activism.

Next, Mark Hannah and Susie Salmon respond to changes to laws regarding insanity plea defenses and the removal of the plea as an affirmative defense that leaves these defendants vulnerable to unjust legal consequences. They do so by outlining a framework for technical communicators to act as intermediaries between support stakeholders such that they might help those stakeholders develop and present arguments that combat stigmas associated with insanity defenses and support defendants' claims that they are not criminally responsible for their actions. Their chapter ultimately explicates how technical communicators from diverse backgrounds can prepare and identify emergent intervention points within a legal case and then later function as coproducers of the law when acting as intermediaries in the support networks.

Likewise, Tianna Cobb examines the stigmatization of mental health and illness within the Black community and beyond. Certain cultural and contextual factors, she argues, have led to the discursive normalization of mental health and illness stigma within the Black community. Yet, the chapter argues, these various discourses are being resisted by community members to destigmatize and promote mental wellness. Presenting a rhetorical autoethnography, Cobb advocates for sharing experiences seeking and getting mental health help in communities where it is especially stigmatized as a strategic intervention into stigma.

This section concludes with Cynthia Ryan's chapter on the concept "anosognosia"—an unawareness of illness status and refusal to seek or accept treatment—via the case of her brother's antisocial personality disorder. A poignant autoethnographic examinations of her experiences living with an abusive family member with severe psychosis, Ryan's chapter breaks new ground in MHRR by intervening in and directly challenging the field's major epistemology—that those labeled "mentally ill" should be ennobled and celebrated for their too-often-ignored rhetorical gifts—to better account for cases of severe psychosis and attendant violence and destruction.

The final section of the book offers pedagogical and cocurricular interventions in three chapters, beginning with Lynn Reid's description of how she sought to combat the stigmas and misinformation surrounding student behavior and mental health through creating a faculty development workshop (in cooperation with her counseling department) that emphasizes scenario-based learning and narrative analysis of selections published on *The Mighty* for an audience of instructors. The goal of these workshops as interventions is to encourage faculty to practice what she calls an "empathy-first approach" when students appear to be disengaged and to recognize that what appears to be disengagement may also reflect sincere mental health struggles that students may not wish to share. The chapter outlines the ways that this workshop sought to function as a method of teaching rhetorical empathy to faculty and gives readers the tools they'll need to adapt the workshop for their own local contexts.

Next, readers will find Leslie Anglesey and Adam Hubrig's suggestions for how to intervene in the rhetorical project that frames the university as mental health champion while placing the onus of mental healthcare on its students, ignoring the institutional roles that sites of postsecondary education play in contributing to and exacerbating anxiety, depression, and other mental health concerns while minimizing a need for institutional change. Anglesey and Hubrig's chapter is followed by Rachel Blasiman and Barbara George's description of the ways narratives can shape how students "read" and engage with online mental health support tools. Seeking to offer others working in higher education useful data through which they might approach mental health support services with their own students, their chapter ultimately explores multiple framing narratives to highlight how these narratives impact student mental health-seeking behaviors and understanding of mental health definitions.

As we hope this introduction has demonstrated, this volume has much to offer a wide range of researchers, activists, and practitioners. Engaging with the rhetorics of mental health as vital considerations for making an impact on the messy object that is mental health, chapter authors offer readers concrete takeaways they can bring to their own MHRR-related projects and initiatives. We hope readers find much value in the methodological; legal, cultural, and institutional; and pedagogical and cocurricular interventions. We do not claim, however, that these interventions are beyond critical reproach. Some might argue that they do too little to stem the tide of new mental illness categories; others might claim that they do not go far enough to address the new and worsening mental health landscape that marks these times of public health crises and racial trauma. It would be easy to also consider some of the work to be giving over too much to medicalized notions of mental health. We do not pretend that such critiques are without merit. Instead, the claim here is that engaging with the rhetorics of mental health is inevitable, that doing so thoughtfully and with the aim of making an impact is necessary, and that this collection is only the beginning of the work that is needed in strategic interventions in mental health rhetoric.

Intervention's etymology shares its origins with invention. Both originate from the Latin *venir*, to come. For intervention, it comes into being in the in-between spaces, in the middle, while invention is simply the act of becoming, of creating. We end with this linguistic twist to highlight how interventions are in fact inventions, ways of coming between to create something new. A collection like this one will always be and has always been relevant. In some ways, then, mental health is the ultimate *kairotic* signifier. Mental health can easily be invoked as an especially timely and essential area of inquiry, and MHRR is but one slice of scholarly terrain that sets out to make sense of its complexity.

We hope the essays in this volume inspire readers to build their own theories, to alter, to adjust, to improve their own practice, and to encourage scholars to consider inventive ways rhetoric can intervene in and create new understandings of mental health rhetorical research.

Note

1 We acknowledge the communication theory rhetoric of social intervention (Brown, 1982). The way we are using "intervention" is narrower than Brown's conception of a systemic framework. We see interventional rhetoric as focusing on specific moments and in smaller contexts (see Melonçon, 2017 for more on smaller contexts) than the Brown's framework.

References

Alvesson, Mats, & Kärreman, Dan. (2011). *Qualitative research and theory development: Mystery as method.* Sage. https://dx.doi.org/10.4135/9781446287859

Brown, William R. (1982). Attention and the rhetoric of social intervention. *Quarterly Journal of Speech, 68*(1), 17–27. doi:10.1080/00335638209383588

Emmons, Kimberly K. (2010). *Black dogs and blue words: Depression and gender in the age of self-care*. Rutgers University Press.

Gorski, P. C. (2019). Fighting racism, battling burnout: Causes of activist burnout in US racial justice activists. *Ethnic and Racial Studies, 42*(5), 667–687. https://doi.org/10.1080/01419870.2018.1439981

Hanganu-Bresch, Christina, & Berkenkotter, Carol. (2019). *Diagnosing madness: The discursive construction of the psychiatric patient, 1850–1920*. University of South Carolina Press. https://doi.org/10.2307/j.ctv7r41gv

Holladay, Drew. (2017). Classified conversations: Psychiatry and tactical technical communication in online spaces. *Technical Communication Quarterly, 26*(1), 8–24. doi:10.1080/10572252.2016.1257744

Kar, Sujita K., Yasir Arafat S. M., Kabir, Russell, Sharma, Pawan, & Saxena, Shailendra K. (2020). Coping with mental health challenges during COVID-19. In S. K. Saxena (Ed.), *Coronavirus disease 2019 (COVID-19): Epidemiology, pathogenesis, diagnosis, and therapeutics* (pp. 199–213). Springer. https://doi.org/10.1007/978-981-15-4814-7_16

Kumar, Anant, & Nayar, Rajasekharan. (2020). COVID 19 and its mental health consequences. *Journal of Mental Health, 30*(1), 1–2. https://doi.org/10.1080/09638237.2020.1757052

Law, John. (2004). *After method: Mess in social science research*. Routledge.

Lyne, John. (2001). Contours of intervention: How rhetoric matters to biomedicine. *Journal of Medical Humanities, 22*(1), 3–13. https://doi.org/10.1023/A:1026622309671

Mahase, Elisabeth. (2020). Covid-19: Mental health consequences of pandemic need urgent research, paper advises. *BMJ, 369*, m1515. https://doi.org/10.1136/bmj.m1515

McCarthy, Lucille P., & Gerring, Joan P. (1994). Revising psychiatry's charter document: DSM-IV. *Written Communication, 11*(2), 147–192. doi:10.1177/0741088394011002001

McKnight-Eily, Lela R., Okoro, Catherine A., Strine, Tara W., Verlenden, Jorge, Hollis, Natasha D., Njai, Rashid, Mitchell, Elizabeth W., Board, Amy, Puddy, Richard, & Thomas, Craig. (2021). Racial and ethnic disparities in the prevalence of stress and worry, mental health conditions, and increased substance use among adults during the Covid-19 pandemic—United states, April and May 2020. *Morbidity and Mortality Weekly Report, 70*(5), 162–166. https://doi.org/10.15585/mmwr.mm7005a3

Melonçon, Lisa. (2017). Patient experience design: expanding usability methodologies for healthcare. *Communication Design Quarterly Review, 5*(2), 19–28. https://dl.acm.org/doi/10.1145/3131201.3131203

Nadal, Kevin L., Griffin, Katie E., Wong, Yinglee, Hamit, Sahran, & Rasmus, Morgan. (2014). The impact of racial microaggressions on mental health: Counseling implications for clients of color. *Journal of Counseling & Development, 92*(1), 57–66. https://doi.org/10.1002/j.1556-6676.2014.00130.x

Ornell, Felipe, Schuch, Jaqueline B., Sordi, Anne O., Kessler, Felix H. P. (2020). "Pandemic fear" and Covid-19: Mental health burden and strategies. *Brazilian Journal of Psychiatry, 42*(3), 232–235. https://doi.org/10.1590/1516-4446-2020-0008

Owens, Kim H. (2015). *Writing childbirth: Women's rhetorical agency in labor and online*. Southern Illinois University Press.

Pereira-Sanchez, Victor, Adiukwu, Frances, Hayek, Samer E., Bytyçi, Drita G., Gonzalez-Diaz, Jairo M., Kundadak, Ganesh K., Larnaout, Amine, Nofal, Marwa, Orsolini, Laura, Ramalho, Rodrigo, Ransing, Ramdas, Shalbafan, Mohammadreza, Soler-Vidal, Joan, Syarif, Zulvia, Teixeira, Andre L. S., & Costa, Mariana

P. (2020). COVID-19 effect on mental health: Patients and workforce. *The Lancet Psychiatry, 7*(6), e29–e30. https://doi.org/10.1016/S2215-0366(20)30153-X

Prendergast, Catherine J. (2001). On the rhetorics of mental disability. In J. C. Wilson & C. Lewiecki-Wilson (Eds.), *Embodied rhetorics: Disability in language and culture* (pp. 45–60). Southern Illinois University Press.

Price, Margaret. (2011). *Mad at school: Rhetorics of mental disability and academic life.* The University of Michigan Press. doi:10.3998/mpub.1612837

Reynolds, J. Fred. (2018). A short history of mental health rhetoric research (MHRR). *Rhetoric of Health and Medicine, 1*(1–2). https://doi.org/10.5744/rhm.2018.1003

Rothfelder, Katy, & Thornton, Davi. (2017). Man interrupted: Mental illness narrative as a rhetoric of proximity. *Rhetoric Society Quarterly, 47*(4), 359–382. doi:10.1080/02 773945.2017.1279343

Scott, J. Blake, & Melonçon, Lisa. (2018). Manifesting methodologies for the rhetoric and health and medicine. In L. Melonçon & J. B. Scott (Eds.), *Methodologies for the rhetoric of health and medicine* (pp. 1–23). Routledge.

Uthappa, N. Renuka. (2017). Moving closer: Speakers with mental disabilities, deep disclosure, and agency through vulnerability. *Rhetoric Review, 36*(2), 164–175. doi:1 0.1080/07350198.2017.1282225

Yergeau, Remi & Huebner, Bryce. (2017). Minding theory of mind. *Journal of Social Philosophy, 48*(3), 273–296. doi:10.1111/josp.12191

PART I
Methodological Interventions

1

A THEORY OF COLLECTIVE INTIMACY

Lisa Melançon and Lora Arduser

As new fields, mental health rhetoric (MHR) and its sister field rhetoric of health and medicine (RHM) have embraced methodological mutability or creative approaches to rethinking methodologies, methods, and theories in ways that are responsive to specific, local projects (Scott and Melançon, 2018). In doing so, the fields have introduced a number of new theories (see, e.g., Bivens, Arduser, Welhausen, & Faris, 2018; Campbell and Angeli, 2019; Kessler, 2020; Melançon, 2018a) to frame research practice and to guide analysis and interpretation of artifacts. We follow this trend—as well as the interventional directive of this volume—to offer a theoretical intervention that can be used as a methodological framework.

Thinking of intervention as an invitation to create new theories and to intervene in existing practices, we offer the theory of "collective intimacy" (defined at length below). Our choice to theory-build has been conceptualized in the RHM chapter: "Theory building' call[s] attention to the act of creating, extending, or adapting theory as an inventional practice and as a key contribution of rhetorical inquiry" (Scott & Gouge, 2019, p. 181; also see Scott & Melançon, 2018). Creating a theory as an inventional practice allows an expansion of rhetorical inquiry such that it might adapt to changes in communication patterns. We illustrate theory-building via "collective intimacy," which is a theory that offers a generative framework for understanding the multiple layers that contribute to communication practices in online health forums. In doing so, we participate in theory-building that "emerge[d] through the challenging of established patterns rather than through attempts to put the bits of the jigsaw back together" (Alvesson & Kärreman, 2011, p. 21).

For the purposes of this chapter, we operationalize online health forums as locations where patients, their families, or caregivers congregate to share

DOI: 10.4324/9781003144854-3

information and find support. We use "online health forum" generically to include sponsored forums from US health organizations (e.g., the American Diabetes Association), patient-sponsored groups (e.g., TuDiabetes), Facebook groups, and communities that form around specific twitter hashtags (e.g., #migraine). RHM scholars have examined such online health forums as research sites (see, e.g., Arduser 2017a, 2017b, 2013, 2011; McCaughey, 2021; Pengilly, 2019).[1] A notable exception is Drew Holladay's (2016) study that examined how writers grapple with mental health diagnostic discourses in online discussion boards. His study is most illuminating in its use of interviews with forum participants. Yet, what is still missing from his and other MHR and RHM literature is a strong methodological apparatus that could help researchers to draw innovative conclusions from studying online health forums.

Likewise, while existing work on health forums is important, we sense that research that focuses on theme spotting or discourse analysis within a singular forum focused on one condition potentially limits scholars' understanding of the relationships between people, information, and technology. In this chapter, therefore, we offer a theoretical framework to analyze and to examine how relationships are being *reconfigured* and *mediated* in multiple online health spaces. Digital technologies have rapidly changed where people engage in information and dialogue exchange. Technologies that enable online health forums help people overcome constraints, such as local cultural norms governing intimacy, as well as logistical barriers to meeting face-to-face or in public. The increased reliance on digital technologies means scholars are having to consider new ways of understanding the relationships that form online because these relationships are more prevalent and are frequently taking place in people's homes. The latter means there is a necessity to understand how the relative privacy of home—a site of intimacy between partners, families, and friends—now also come to be sites of intimacy between relative strangers. To examine this tension in the rest of this chapter, we offer an extended definition of collective intimacy as a theory that draws attention to the complex ontologies of online health forums and offers ways that rhetorical scholars in RHM and MHR can consider using this theory in their own work.

Theory Building in MHR and RHM

RHM scholars have long looked at online discourse as a research site and information in online spaces as research artifacts to understand communication practices around different health conditions (see, e.g., Arduser, 2017b, 2013; de Hertogh, 2015; McKinley, 2019). However, the nature of most of those investigations are looking at a single site and, therefore, provide one-dimensional insights into a narrow realm of the particular forum. For example, Katrina Hinson's (2016) analysis of a Facebook group of people who suffered a venous thrombolytic event confirmed many of the same findings as other studies on online health forums. That is, Hinson claimed that the group helped to transform the participants, while also helping others through eliciting empathy, sharing experiences, and developing a platform upon which to critique health-care practices. These insights are important, yet more work is needed to deepen the conclusions that can be drawn from examining such research sites.

The same problems hold true in MHR. Recent work specific to mental health online forums has pointed to some limitations of current research approaches. For example, health communication researcher Jesse W. C. Yip (2020) argued that content analysis—the primary research method for examining online forums—can no longer stand alone to understand emotional and informational support for those who post on mental health forums. Yip claimed mixed methods approaches were needed, where Holladay's (2017) work can be taken as an example. As another MHR example, psychologist Julie Prescott and colleagues Terry Hanley and Katalin Ujhelyi (2017) confirmed previous research that online health forums are helpful for young people and their mental health. Their contribution was gaining insights into the types of approaches (directive or nondirective) used for support within the forum, but by their own admission, their findings likely have little relevance outside of the forum itself. What current research in RHM, rhetoric, and other fields do have in common in regard to looking at online health forums is the highly focused examination of the textual as a way to understand the patient perspective through their language. We argue that this approach, while valuable in uncovering patients' vernacular approaches to health literacies, still leave many questions unanswered about context and material conditions at the backdrop of the posts and, more particularly, about the relationship of people, information, and technologies. Importantly, such studies leave scholars needing additional ways to make sense of information across forums and to consider communication dimensions outside of the isolation of one particular context.

Sanna Malinen's (2015) systematic review of empirical studies of user participation in online communities found that in the spite of the "large amount of research conducted on the topic [of online communities], a theoretical and conceptual framework for user participation remains undefined as most of the research has approached participation in terms of its quantity" (p. 228). As scholars know, the power and benefit of theory is that it provides alternative ways to understand a phenomenon, and without new theories, scholarship risks stagnating. What MHR and RHM need, then, is to develop ways of extending our analytic techniques to gain deeper and more extensive ways of examining online heath forums. A key role of theory building around online health forums is to address Malinen's concern and implicit call for more nuanced approaches. Research in RHM and MHR and in related fields have studied online health forums through the lens of communities (Beemer, 2016; King, 2017; Lian & Grue, 2017; Willis, 2016; Willis & Royne, 2017). Some studies, such as Lora Arduser's (2011), take community a step further and examine ways the forum members describe their experiences. Our goal with building out our term "collective intimacy" is to advance the approach Arduser (2011) took in trying to understand online health forums outside of a singular community framework.

While such studies do provide insight into how patients communicate, examining forums in isolation does not actually help scholars understand how the forums function. Rather, the intense focus on the discourses within the forum seems to gloss over what the forums may actually be able to tell researchers about their function. That is, there are consequences for the *form* of the discourse within the forums. Creating new theories or new conceptual apparatus to understand those consequences is a key goal for scholars in rhetoric and in RHM. In other words, community and the existing scholarship on it does not adequately provide a theoretical mechanism to fully uncover the dynamics of relationships across and between multiple communities.

More so, moving beyond community as a descriptor or characteristic of why people gather allows deeper insights into why people continue to connect in these spaces. While existing research certainly lays a strong foundation for understanding online health forums, the evolution of online health forums now requires scholars to go one step farther, to move toward new interventions. Thinking of the collection's focus on "interventions" as providing an imperative to make an impact leads us to consider it as inherently inventional. That is, we see "interventions" in relation to rhetorical methodologies for studying online health forums as providing us with a space to think through what is needed to impact and advance this area of inquiry. Our response is that theory-building is needed to intervene effectively in established communities of research practice, and our specific intervention—our theory "collective intimacy"—provides an example of how new theories promise to fundamentally shift research practice in highly generative ways.

In the next section, we build the theory of collective intimacy to both show how theory building can be an intervention into an established set of practices and to provide an intervention into the routinized research practices surrounding rhetoric and/of online health forums. This theory of collective intimacy becomes the basis for rethinking the relationship between humans, technology, and information as experienced in online health forums. Conceptual and theoretical distinctions and dimensions matter in how we view discourses, primarily patient and caregiver discourses, in online forums. The vulnerability of the moment when someone is moved to participate in an online health forum—the need for a different type of relationship from language—means that we need different theoretical orientations to fully understand the dimensions, affect, and ramifications of these sites. The theory and subsequent examination of existing scholarship provides RHM scholars to move toward answering more complex questions about the role and importance of patient-to-patient (or peer-to-peer) information exchange.

Collective Intimacy

When we were considering how to describe the theory we envisioned, we needed a descriptor before "intimacy." Since "intimacy" is so readily associated with personal relationships, we wanted to signal that this form of intimacy was somewhat different than this traditional form. We settled on "collective" because it encapsulates two important features of the theoretical construct we are building.

First, "collective" invokes a sense of the cumulative. In her analysis of video logs of trans YouTube creators, Laura Horak (2014) claimed that "there is a strong formal similarity from one vlog to the next" and that "the cumulative force of these statements of presence draw upon each other to establish community" (p. 581). In the same way, words, phrases, themes, and tropes repeat across various health forums (i.e., vlogs, online forums) in ways that accumulate and help to establish the wider community of everyday health information and support-seeking as it unfolds online. This collective and the accumulation of its key features become a collection worth further examination, which is vital if scholarship is going to move from forum to forum and channel to channel because it conceptualizes a collective that brings together individual experiences and gathers those same experiences into a communal voice.

Second, the term "collective" also signals cooperation between and among participants in specific health forums and within the larger community of online health forums in general. The emphasis on cooperation provides a foundation of trust and predictability on which intimacy can build and grow; the emphasis on connection invokes that which is necessary for any relationship to become intimate—the ability for disparate parties to find ways to associate and relate to one another in fundamental ways. Such things are highly important to the lives of those who participate. Thus, "collective" and these various connotations help us to flesh out what we mean by a "collective intimacy."

In putting forward our theory, we are also aware that intimacy has not been a term that has been used a great deal as a theoretical apparatus. A notable exception is Shaka McGlotten (2013), who tracked "technologically mediated intimacies" (p. 9) in queer spaces online. McGlotten's complementary work helped us to consider the import and force that intimacy and expanded definitions of what intimacy could mean. McGlotten insisted that "intimacy wasn't something to be captured, but something to be experienced as the pressure, ephemerality, and multiplicity of desire" (McGlotten, p. 22). For our purposes, McGlotten's emphasis on intimacy as something to be experienced helped us expand more traditional definitions that consider intimacy to be something of a personal or private nature (Merriam Webster). Rather, the internet and the myriad options through social media mean that there is an ongoing blurring or fluctuation between private and public (Arduser, 2017b), which now arguably exist on a continuum of experiences where people negotiate daily and even hourly what it means to be public or private or semi-public. Of course, the enormous increase of online communication as a replacement for face-to-face interactions in the context of the COVID-19 pandemic accelerated this movement to much more complex conceptualizations of the public, the private, and the liminal. This ever-expanding purview of the continuum of public-ness also brings with it other questions that were once only the purview of the private, including our notion of what defines intimacy.

Like many other concepts, intimacy, too, is typically socially constructed. Even though intimacy has been traditionally considered that which occurs between those people with whom someone has a close face-to-face relationship, Yi-Fu Tuan (1986) suggested that strangers are an infinite source of possibility for connection, inspiration, and renewal and that we all start out as strangers in any relationship. The movement from stranger to something else highlights the dichotomy of public and private. Our interest in tracking the public and private in relation to intimacy led us to rely on Lauren Berlant (1998) and her conceptualization of intimacy as occurring through contradictory awareness of private and proximate and distant and close, which are also related to online spaces.

Specifically, the idea that intimacy is not fixed and is "portable, unattached to concrete space" and in fact is the "drive that creates spaces around it" (Berlant, 1998, p. 284) helps us to capture what we mean by collective intimacy because of the somewhat paradoxical idea that intimate relationships can start with strangers in public rather than close contacts in private settings. The idea of "public" and "private" has been discussed in rhetorical scholarship, particularly with the rise of the internet and its disruptions in traditional conceptions of space. For example, Barbara Couture (2004) laid out the stakes of blending public rhetoric and private lives, while Sidney Dobrin (2004) argued that distinctions between public and private discourses actually limit understanding of communication practices. These rhetorical considerations that the distinctions between public and private are not necessarily generative complement Berlant in that they forcefully underscore how intimacy can bring together two realms often thought to be separate, that "what makes a public sphere intimate is an expectation that the consumers of its particular stuff *already* share a worldview and emotional knowledge that they have derived from a broadly common historical experience…" (Berlant, 2008, p. viii). Participants in online health forums, thus, bring their experiences into a new space searching for an intimate connection. There is an intimacy with one's illness or chronic condition that is inescapable. There is also an intimacy between people who share the same condition or problem. There is an intimacy in sharing the emotional toll of experiencing and managing care in complex healthcare systems that often are not designed with the patient in mind.

In online health forums, the intimacy is capitalized as a means to building trust within the relationship(s) with other participants. The collective also highlights how "intimacy works as an important currency within social media; thus, intimacy can be capitalized in manifold and intersecting ways, for example, for monetary purposes, social recognition and as a tool in advocacy work" (Raun, 2018, p. 101). Posts and discussions become an intimate currency meant to establish more than simply a common ground and a common experience. Rather, the discourse becomes an extension of the most vulnerable and hidden self and a leap of faith that this vulnerability will be acknowledged and supported rather than dismissed or mocked.

One of the most intimate things that people do is to let others see them at their worst, their most vulnerable, the moments where they feel "not normal." The online forum is "intimate" in that it "foregrounds affective and emotional attachments located in fantasies of the common, the everyday, and a sense of ordinariness, a space where the social world is rich with anonymity and local recognitions....It is textually mediated" (Berlant, 2008, p. 10). When patients and family members and others visit online forums, they are exposing themselves in an intimate way by allowing others to see them at their lowest, at their weakest, at their most vulnerable moments. It is during those times that true intimacy happens; where there is shared experience when everything is wrong, the most intimate moments occur. And that intimacy happens regularly in online environments between people who are bound together in a collective intimacy based on shared concerns and vulnerability and the need to get information.

In addition to vulnerability, collective intimacy enacts a belonging where participants can "take things in and sometimes circulate what they hear" or "they do not have to do anything to belong. They can be passive and lurk" (Berlant, 2011, p. 227). The multiple roles of participants in online discourse have long been examined. From the power participant who posts all the time to those who simply lurk, there remains intimate space for all participants. Beyond shared interests in the content, moreover, intimacy is enhanced and implemented through a closeness and connection that does not rely on proximity. Rather, intimacy comes into being through a sense of emotional connection over something shared that is not tied to anything except the sense of belonging and related to someone else who is experiencing or feeling the same things. Sasha Roseneil and Shelley Budgeon (2004) opened up family to move beyond the traditional notions of familial relations and instead focus on the fact that intimacy and care takes place within networks of friends that extend beyond partners and immediate biological family connections. Shifting conceptions of social norms and who qualifies as family expands not only the people with which intimacy can occur but also the locations where intimacy can take place. Intimacy is about trust and truth. Within this expanded notion of family, certain personal—intimate—information can be shared in more and more places. These forums allow users to stand exposed and vulnerable; the forum participants embrace that exposure and vulnerability with a safety and assurance.

The space where vulnerability and assurance meet is an intimate truth. And it is important to bring into view how online places can enable intimacy, particularly around issues that carry a sense of stigma such as mental health.

Collective intimacy functions because one needs to live within a particular personal situation and draws on the collective community for support and knowledge. In this way, "a certain circularity structures an intimate public" as "its consumer participants are perceived to be marked by a commonly lived history; its narratives and things are deemed expressive of that history *while also shaping its conventions of belonging*" (Berlant, 2008, p. viii, emphasis added). Even with all of these nuances articulated, it should be noted that intimate publics, and the way that we are using intimacy here is not radically different from its usual definition. However, we are shifting the way intimacy is applied as a theoretical construct. We want to shift it from something usually considered as private to something public (as in Berlant's use). We also want to emphasize that intimacy is not confined to one-on-one relationships, where collective intimacy can bring multiple participants together toward a common aim. This is a minor, yet important distinction in understanding the role of online health forums as a form of collective intimacy and more so in understanding the important of collective intimacy as a way to understand how communication circulation and knowledge building happens in health contexts. In making these distinctions, we are doing much of what Berlant (1998) asked: "To rethink intimacy is to appraise how we have been and how we live and how we might imagine lives that make more sense than the ones so many are living" (p. 286), and imagining different lives is what so many who participate in online health forums are searching for.

Collective intimacy is thus defined as a cooperative relationship between and among multiple participants around a common topic or concern that is usually tied to a personal experience that makes one feel vulnerable. Collective intimacy, moreover, has the following characteristics: distributed, relational, and affective. We discuss these characteristics in the next section as a way to offer an extended definition of the term.

Characteristics

We wanted to consider the parts, the characteristics, of collective intimacy outside of our use of collective and our interpretation of intimacy. These characteristics clarify ways other scholars can descriptively use the theory to understand the relationship between technology and information. By providing characteristics to be diversely interpreted, scholars can use these to analyze dimensions of communication. In other words, they give others an immediate heuristic to start their own investigations into online health forums. The three main characteristics that create a collective intimacy are: distributed, relational, and affective.

Distributed

We offer this first characteristic to address what may be an immediate concern— the potentially contradictory interpretation of "collective" as aligned to "distributed." While paradoxical on the surface, the two ideas actual align quite well. Collective refers to the intimate nature of the discourse and the potency of multiple participants' experiences and knowledge, while distributed attends to the physical locations of those participants. Distributed allows scholars to account for the dispersed nature of communication across platforms, time, and space, while taking into account the embodied distribution of the participants themselves.

Online health forums extend locations and spaces where communication about health and medicine take place. It's not simply that the forum helps to bring people together for a variety of reasons; it literally expands, extends and distributes where the communication can take place. In putting forth distributed as a key characteristic of collective intimacy, we follow Andre Brock (2020) who argued for *distributed* to mean a "holistic approach to analyzing technology as discourse, practice, and artifact" (p. 2). Rather than simply accepting distributed as a way to account for the physical distances and distribution of people who post in online health forums, Brock urged scholars to think in more nuanced ways. By expanding distributed to fully implicate technology as practice and artifact allows researchers to think through the importance of technology in creating intimate spaces and relationships. The incorporation of distributed as a key component of the theory and its definition also works as a potentially generative form of encounter that technology facilitates.

Distributed also connects with recent moves in rhetorical scholarship on circulation, "conceived here in terms of spatiotemporal flow as well as a cultural-rhetorical process" (Gries, 2018, p. 3). Circulation expands the rhetorical canon of delivery to make explicit the movement of texts and ideas within a community. In this sense, the distributed nature of collective intimacy enters into these conversations by emphasizing how the same concerns of online forum participants play out across different forums or different technological platforms. In other words, if one were to trace the circulation of an idea between and among different online health forums, scholars would gain a deeper sense of the impact of that idea's distribution. Thus, distributed as a characteristic of collective intimacy can "cultivate new understanding about how rhetoric unfolds and acquires force in an increasingly digitally networked and globalized world" (Gries, 2018, p. 8).

The distributed characteristic of collective intimacy has a temporal dimension as well as a tie to space and circulation. Online health forums disrupt the typical, linear conception of time since participants can log on and participate at any given time. Distributed takes into account the dual temporalities of online health forums. They are both immediate (whenever a participant logs on) and archival (remains online even after information is posted). Temporality is then distributed and non-linear (Melonçon, 2018b).

While we definitely came upon collective intimacy because of technology and online forums, we've come to realize that the idea of collective intimacy and the characteristic of distributed works in other locations as well. That is, distribution can be mobile as seen in Augustine's (this collection) examination of the paratherapeutic process for those who experienced domestic violence or the knitting events for postpartum mothers in China facilitated by social media (see Wang in this collection). These examples point to diverse ways that the distributed nature of bringing people together in collectives is important for RHM and MHR scholars to consider.

Relational

We turn to relational here to highlight relationships between people, technology, and information that lead to the formation of the collective. A focus on the relational "help[s] remind us that a relationship is not a discrete, state entity but rather a process of the interaction of forces" (Condit, 2010, p. 6). Relational forces play an important role in the development of intimate connections as "intimacy is supported by a range of discourses and practices, but as an experience it is composed largely of feelings, feeling more or less connected, as if one belongs or doesn't" (McGlotten, 2013, p. 9). Intimacy is developed because much of the information shared online in forums is about stories, reaching out, and being supported. In short, intimacy is created through sharing, observing, learning, discovery, friendship, and most of all, a mutual engagement around a common issue or problem.

Importantly, relationalities are often built on participants' intentionally partial versions of self. As Jeff Grabill and Stacy Pigg (2012) observed, "given the nature of most online interactions, participants often do not build fully formed or coherent portraits of who they are as people, but rather draw on parts of their identity to accomplish other goals within the conversation" (p. 102). This limiting of identity can reveal itself in intimate ways. Through collective intimacy, these partial identity constructions can still hold value as markers in understanding what parts of an identity are key to sharing the lived experiences of illness in ways that help to form relationships with other people.

Relationships and their interactions, too, are all dependent on social roles and behaviors, and most particularly on how the particular individual interacts with others. Collective intimacy and its relational characteristic also take into account the numerous people involved in health care. Take the caregiver who is often caring for a spouse or parent or a child. There is an intimacy in that relationship that moves from the familial relationship to the healthcare relationship. This concept, which can be seen in Sean Kamperman's notion of inclusive tactics (this volume), also highlights the relational capacity of collective intimacy. Scholars need to "rethink intimacy" because any attempt to theorize multiple simultaneous instantiations of conversations within an online forum (or a group setting) needs a way to articulate the relationship between those instantiations. The relational characteristic is the beginning step to move from individuals to a collective, and it intersects with the circulation aspect of distribution by providing boundaries to relationships.

Collective intimacy is a way to form relationships with others as a means of care and well-being. For those people who engage in online spaces, there is a desire for a relationship, an intimacy, which cannot be found in other spaces and locations or filled by other people in their lives. Social media scholars have found that, in some cases, the relationships people have online can be as real as those they have face-to-face. What makes the health and medical relationship different from most online communities that grow out of non-medical issues and topics is the level of intimacy because of the embodied nature of the interactions and information that is shared.

Affect

The final characteristic of collective intimacy is affect. In the recent "affective turn," scholars (see, e.g., Anderson, 2009; Leys, 2011; Wetherell, 2014) have emphasized different affective dimensions as a way to think through the co-creation of meaning that is embodied and material. Affect moves into writing studies from cultural studies, which define affect as something almost mystical, such as an intensity (Massumi, 2002), or as a vital force (Seigworth and Gregg, 2010). Trying to put the intensity and force into the everyday, we want to highlight the embodied dimension of affect.

We use affect as a distinctly human and embodied theoretical orientation. Unlike some theorists who have invoked affect in a more material way that dehumanizes the human, we want to prioritize the human. Indeed, "affect is found in those intensities that pass body to body...in those resonances that circulate about, between, and sometimes stick to bodies and world" (Seigworth & Gregg, 2010, p. 1). The passing of body to body is an intimate act, and ensuring that scholars do not lose sight of the physical bodies that enact this intimacy is a key reason to include affect as a characteristic of collective intimacy.

Affect enables the theory of collective intimacy to gain force through accounting for the wide range of affective, embodied modes found in forums. From helplessness to empowerment and from isolation to community, affect, which is already theorized in some ways, gives a needed dimension in gaining insights into the reasons and rationales for the creation, growth, and continued participation in forums. Online forums provide "encounters with others" that leave participants "affected—moved or changed by a feeling or an emotion in relation to someone or something"; they also highlight the fact that "we are always open to some degree to being affected by the emotional-evaluative stance that others take towards us" (Burkitt, 2014, p. 169). Affect is meditated through technologies in online health forums; using affect as a lens helps account for how participants make sense out of the emotional freight of health and medical conditions, both chronic and acute.

Online spaces are, thus, examples of affective landscapes of care: examination of the discourses in these spaces afford scholars the opportunity to know how technical spaces impact care, lived experiences of health and illness, and quality of life. In these spaces, "belonging is made of the affective or material ties and obligations that link the individuals to others" (McGlotten, 2013, p. 22). Importantly, too, participation in these landscapes of care produce affective engagements that illustrate the way "patients" live their everyday lives. This information offers scholars the opportunity to study ways to better communicate and engage patients and caregivers; it, likewise, offers practitioners the opportunity to create health and medical communication that is actually useful to patients and caregivers.

Using affect as a key component of a theoretical lens reorients how to rhetorically analyze the discourse in online spaces because affect calls to mind the embodied dimensions of participants. Since "knowledge cannot be separated from the bodily world of feeling and sensation" (Ahmed, 2004, p. 171), an affective characteristic is necessary for understanding participants in online health forums and is equally valuable in examining the researcher's own positionality. Collective intimacy and its affect characteristic, then, might offer additional insights to complement Tianna Cobb's autoethnographic explication of Black women's mental health (in this collection).

The theory of collective intimacy we have described in this chapter—distributed, relational, and affective—offers a way to understand how people make sense of their health and illnesses in online spaces beyond examining a single forum and users' discursive practices therein. It also gives us a theoretical way to closely examine the rhetorical constructions found in these spaces. Scholars in RHM and MHR are in need of new ways to make sense of novel and ongoing experiences of the participants in online health forums. Collective intimacy's characteristics can help provide a framework through which these everyday health and medical spaces can be tracked or coded and, thus, adds to our ability to understand online health forums and the participants a bit better. The characteristics of collective intimacy and their definitions—as well as the construct itself—are meant as a starting place, and we offer collective intimacy to RHM and MHR scholars to inspire new and more expansive work in this area. We want others to refine, to expand, or to contradict the ideas we put forward here as we work to collectively understand the world of health and medicine better via the potential of rhetoric as an analytic device. Since mental health is, as the introduction to this volume argues, a particularly complex and fraught health and medical area, collective intimacy might be an especially generative theoretical framework for inquiries in mental health rhetoric.

Conclusion and Future Research Directions

Focusing on theory-building for richer inquiries in online health forums in mental health and beyond, this chapter has provided an expanded definition of collective intimacy and its characteristics: distributed, relational, and affective. As a new term, it participates in the theory-building work necessary for scholars to see phenomenon differently and to draw new and distinctive conclusions that can help improve understanding. Collective intimacy is, likewise, a theoretical framework from which scholars might adequately analyze the discourses found online. It underscores the innate need of people to make substantial and meaningful attachments. Those attachments, as we have shown, do not have to be in person or even with people that are known to them. Collective intimacy, then, accounts for the need and desire to form attachments to others, as elaborated by Martha Nussbaum (2001) as essential to well-being (p. 79). Ultimately, this theory affords a way to interrogate an ontological perspective of what intimacy means for the relationship between people, information, and technology. Collective intimacy allows for a deeper understanding of the intimate connections made between relative strangers that rely on set of a characteristics that a community together, intimately. Shifting from singular to collective experiences emphasizes the relational capacities between people that are distributed across time and space.

As both theory and methodology, distributed intimacy provides a framework that helps scholars do four things. First, following the intimate traces no matter how distributed allow researchers to gain insights into not only how these intimate connections are established but also into how they might leverage understandings into patient (and caregiver) experiences in ways that account for time, space, technologies, and bodies. The characteristics of collective intimacy afford scholars the opportunity to expand our tools for understanding community formations and what holds them together or breaks them apart; it adds additional tools for rhetorical analysis of health discourse, and for gaining insights into how to improve the creation of communication interventions.

Second, with a theory of collective intimacy, researchers can begin to see how the affective connection actually intervenes into the communication process and then theoretically, researchers can track what happens next, particularly in terms of how intimacy relates to decision-making. Researchers are just now beginning to understand such relational aspects of online health forums. Without these sorts of new ways of researching forums, we limit ourselves to a series of unconnected studies that do not advance our understanding of language and persuasion in forums outside of the isolated and narrow view of theme or pattern spotting in singular forums. We hope this theory and its examination across different illness forums will help us understand the ongoing struggles for meaning not only around an illness but also in terms of the reflection of the everydayness of living with a disease (either chronic or otherwise).

Third, collective intimacy gives insights and deeper understanding to the private, to the public, to the collective, and to the personal. It is the connective tissue between and among people. So of course, intimacy should be a driving characteristic of the next generation of online discourse research. This relational sharing provides scholars in mental health rhetoric, and rhetoric more broadly, additional tools to gain insights into how information is mediated and circulated online.

Finally, we see collective intimacy as a way to move RHM and MHR beyond a singular focus on thematic discourse analysis toward work that promises to contribute to more theory-building. Indeed,

> theory is often seen as providing direction and control, but it can also be mobilized as a tool for disclosure. A theory can open up not only other theories and their lines of interpretation but also sensitive constructions and interpretations.
>
> *(Alvesson & Kärreman, 2011, p. 37)*

Researchers cannot intervene and offer suggestions to improve practice or policy (or anything) without a more in-depth understanding of how patients and their families negotiate their illnesses in the everyday settings of their lives, including in online forums.

To move this type of research forward, we offer some immediate questions for other scholars to consider. While much of our chapter offers the extended explication of how we understand collective intimacy, these questions constitute something of a heuristic for immediate use as scholars attempt to make use of, extend, challenge, and refine this term:

- What is the relationship between place and technology?
- How might technology be interrogated specifically through the lens of collective intimacy?
- How is intimacy produced in spaces, and how does it move (can it actually be used as a true testable theory)?
- How does intimacy and related knowledge circulate and relate to subjectivities and the material body?
- Are there particular places and spaces that are invested in intimacy, and what is the lived experience because of that?
- What can a theory of intimacy show us about the importance of online forums and discourses?
- How is intimacy productive of spaces?
- Do intimacy theories help us with understanding the contradictions and the binaries that are often found in these spaces? How does it help us understand participants' willingness and desire to both relate and reckon?

- What new insights might scholars learn if collective intimacy works alongside considerations of classical rhetorical terms and concepts such as Eudaimonia, metis, hexis, phusis, and kairos (to name but a few)?

Collective intimacy is a theoretical affective structure that can be used as an interpretative framework for discourse across different types and kinds of online forums. It can open ways to theoretically investigate commonalities that can potentially help researchers not only understand what users gain from forums but also help create different types of interventions that may be usefully applied or work toward improving or changing behaviors. In other words, collective intimacy enacts rhetoric's possibility (see, e.g., Boyle, 2018; Poulakos, 1999) as a means to provide another way of seeing, of experiencing relationships. In RHM and MHR, collective intimacy is needed as an alternative to understand that beyond discursive analyses of themes in online forums, there is a need to examine how and why deeply meaningful relationships can occur between people who may not otherwise interact. When scholars find existing interpretative or theoretical lenses not enough, it becomes necessary to innovate and create new ways. Collective intimacy is our attempt to expand possibilities. That said, it is intentionally partial and primed for creative uses beyond our own description of the term. We invite other scholars to use this term in their own work in ways that will evolve and expand its capabilities.

Note

1 Readers will note that we are intentionally limiting our discussion of scholarship confining our citational practice to work more specific to rhetorical studies rather than moving into the vast literature on online health forums from fields beyond rhetoric, writing, and communication since our methodological intervention is meant to be rhetorical in nature.

References

Ahmed, Sara. (2004). *The cultural politics of emotion.* Routledge.

Alvesson, Mats, & Kärreman, Dan. (2011). *Qualitative research and theory development: Mystery as method.* Sage.

Anderson, Ben. (2009). Affective atmospheres. *Emotion, Space and Society, 2*(2), 77–81. doi:10.1016/j.emospa.2009.08.005

Arduser, Lora. (2011). Warp and weft: Weaving the discussion threads of an online community. *Journal of Technical Writing and Communication, 41*(1), 5–31. doi:10.2190/TW.41.1.b

Arduser, Lora. (2013). The care and feeding of the D-Beast: Metaphors of the lived experience of diabetes. In Lisa Melonçon (Ed.), *Rhetorical accessibility: At the intersection of technical communication and disability studies* (pp. 95–113). Routledge.

Arduser, Lora. (2017a). *Living Chronic: Agency and Expertise in the Rhetoric of Diabetes.* Ohio State University Press.

Arduser, Lora. (2017b). Remediating diagnosis: A familiar narrative form or emerging digital genre? In Caroiyn R. Miller & Ashley Rose Kelly (Eds.), *Emerging genres in new media environments* (pp. 63–78). Palgrave/Macmillan.

Beemer, Cristy. (2016). From the margins of healthcare: De-mythicizing cancer online. *Pietho, 19*(1), 92–127.

Berlant, Lauren. (1998). Intimacy: Special issue. *Critical Inquiry, 24*(2), 281–288.

Berlant, Lauren. (2008). *The female complaint: The unfinished business of sentimentality in American culture.* Duke University press.

Berlant, Lauren. (2011). *Cruel Optimism.* Duke University Press.

Bivens, Kristin Marie, Arduser, Lora, Welhausen, Candice A., & Faris, Michael J. (2018). A multisensory literacy approach to biomedical healthcare technologies: Aural, tactile, and visual layered health literacies. *Kairos, 22*(2).

Boyle, Casey. (2018). *Rhetoric as posthuman practice.* Ohio State University Press.

Brock, Jr. Andre. (2020). *Distributed Blackness: African American Cybercultures.* New York University Press.

Burkitt, Ian. (2014). *Emotions and social relations.* Sage.

Campbell, Lillian, & Angeli, Elizabeth L. (2019). Embodied healthcare intuition: A taxonomy of sensory cues used by healthcare providers. *Rhetoric of Health and Medicine, 2*(4), 353–383.

Condit, Celeste. (2010). Communication as relationality. In Gregory J. Shepher, Jeffrey St. John, & Ted Striphas (Eds.), *Communication as…perspectives on theory* (pp. 3–12). Sage.

Couture, Barbara. (2004). Reconciling private lives and public rhetoric: What's at stake? In Barbara Couture & Thomas Kent (Eds.), *The private, the public, and the published: Reconciling private lives and public rhetoric* (pp. 1–16). Utah State University Press.

De Hertogh, Lori Beth. (2015). Reinscribing a new normal: Pregnancy, disability, and health 2.0 in the online natural birthing community, Birth Without Fear. *Ada: A Journal of Gender, New Media, and Technology, 7.*

Dobrin, Sidney. (2004). Going public: Locating public/private discourse. In Barbara Couture & Thomas Kent (Eds.), *The private, the public, and the published: Reconciling Private Lives and Public Rhetoric* (pp. 216–229). Utah State University Press.

Grabill, Jeffrey T., & Pigg, Stacey. (2012). Messy rhetoric: Identity performance as rhetorical agency in online public forums. *Rhetoric Society Quarterly, 42*(2), 99–119. doi:10.1080/02773945.2012.660369

Gries, Laurie E. (2018). Introduction: Circulation as an emerging threshold concept. In Laurie E. Gries & Colin Gifford Brooke (Eds.), *Circulation, writing, & rhetoric* (pp. 3–24). Utah State University Press.

Hinson, Katrina. (2016). Framing illness through facebook enabled online support groups. *Communication Design Quarterly, 4*(2), 22–32.

Holladay, Drew. (2017). Classified conversations: Psychiatry and tactical technical communication in online spaces. *Technical Communication Quarterly, 26*(1), 8–24. doi:10.1080/10572252.2016.1257744

Horak, Laura. (2014). Trans on youtube: Intimacy, visibility, temporality. *TSQ: Transgender Studies Quarterly, 1*(4), 572–585.

Kessler, Molly Margaret. (2020). The ostomy multiple: Toward a theory of rhetorical enactments. *Rhetoric of Health & Medicine, 3*(3), 293–319.

King, Carie S. T. (2017). *The rhetoric of breast cancer: Patient-to-patient discourse in an online community.* Lexington Health Series.

Leys, Ruth. (2011). The turn to affect: A critique. *Critical Inquiry, 37*, 434–472.

Lian, Olaug S., & Grue, Jan. (2017). Generating a social movement online community through an online discourse: The case of myalgic encephalomyelitis. *Journal of Medical Humanities, 38*(2), 173–189. doi:10.1007/s10912-016-9390-8

Malinen, Sanna. (2015). Understanding user participation in online communities: A systematic literature review of empirical studies. *Computers in Human Behavior, 46*, 228–238. doi:10.1016/j.chb.2015.01.004

Massumi, Brian. (2002). *Parables of the virtual: Movement, affect, sensation.* Duke University Press.

McCaughey, Jessica. (2021). The rhetoric of online exclusive pumping communities: Tactical technical communication as eschewing judgment. *Technical Communication Quarterly, 30*(1), 34–47.

McGlotten, Shaka. (2013). *Virtual intimacies: Media, affect, and queer sociality.* State University of New York Press.

McKinley, Marissa. (2019). Analyzing PCOS discourses: Strategies for unpacking chronic illness and taking action. In Jamie Siegel Finer White-Farnham, Bryna & Cathryn Molloy (Eds.), *Women's health advocacy; rhetorical ingenuity for the 21st century* (pp. 34–44). Routledge.

Melançon, Lisa. (2018a). Bringing the body back through performative phenomenology. In Lisa Melançon & J. Blake Scott (Eds.), *Methodologies for the Rhetoric of Health and Medicine* (pp. 96–114). Routledge.

Melançon, Lisa. (2018b, November 29). *Embodied temporality: Expanding kairos.* Hutton Lecture Series. Purdue University.

Nussbaum, Martha C. (2001). *Women and human development: The capabilities approach.* Cambridge University Press.

Pengilly, Cynthia. (2019). Rhetorics of empowerment for managing lupus pain: Patient to patient knowledge sharing in online health forums. In Jamie Siegel Finer White-Farnham, Bryna & Cathryn Molloy (Eds.), *Women's health advocacy; Rhetorical ingenuity for the 21st century* (pp. 45–58). Routledge.

Poulakos, John. (1999). Toward a sophistic definition of rhetoric. In John L. Lucaites, Celeste Condit, & Sally Caudill (Eds.), *Contemporary Rhetorical Theory: A Reader* (pp. 25–34). Guilford Press.

Prescott, Julie, Hanley, Terry, & Ujhelyi, Katalin. (2017). Peer communication in online mental health forums for young people: Directional and nondirectional support. *JMIR Mental Health, 4*(3), 1–12.

Raun, Tobias. (2018). Capitalizing intimacy: New subcultural forms of micro-celebrity strategies and affective labour on YouTube. *Convergence, 24*(1), 99–113. doi:10.1177/1354856517736983

Roseneil, Sasha, & Budgeon, Shelley. (2004). Cultures of intimacy and care beyond 'the family': Personal life and social change in the early 21st century. *Current Sociology, 52*(2), 135–159.

Scott, J. Blake, & Gouge, Catherine. (2019). Theory building in the rhetoric of health & medicine. In Andrea Aldren, Kendall Gerdes, Judy Holiday, & Ryan Skinnell (Eds.), *Reinventing (with) theory in rhetoric and writing studies: Essays in honor of Sharon Crowley* (pp. 181–195). University Press of Colorado and Utah State University Press.

Scott, J. Blake, & Melançon, Lisa. (2018). Manifesting methodologies for the rhetoric and health and medicine. In Lisa Melançon & J. Blake Scott (Eds.), *Methodologies for the rhetoric of health and medicine* (pp. 1–23). Routledge.

Seigworth, Gregory J., & Gregg, Melissa. (2010). An inventory of shimmers. In Melissa Gregg & Gregory J. Seigworth (Eds.), The affect theory reader (pp. 1–25). Duke University Press.

Tuan, Yi-Fu. (1986). Strangers and strangeness. *Geographical Review, 76*(1), 10–19.

Wetherell, Margaret. (2014). Trends in the turn to affect: A social psychological critique. *Body & Society, 21*(2), 139–166. doi:10.1177/1357034x14539020

Willis, Erin. (2016). Patients' self-efficacy within online health communities: Facilitating chronic disease self-management behaviors through peer education. *Health Communication, 31*(3), 299–307. doi:10.1080/10410236.2014.950019

Willis, Erin, & Royne, Marla B. (2017). Online health communities and chronic disease self-management. *Health Communication, 32*(3), 269–278. doi:10.1080/1041023 6.2016.1138278

Yip, Jesse W. C. (2020). Evaluating the communication of online social support: A mixed-methods analysis of structure and content. *Health Communication, 35*(110), 1210–1218.

2

REFLECTIONS ON RESEARCH AS IT UNFOLDS

Inclusive Tactics as a Methodological Intervention

Sean Kamperman

In disability and mental health rhetoric research (MHRR), questions persist about best practices for including the voices and perspectives of vulnerable participants in the research process. Researchers must weigh the benefits and drawbacks of a range of methodological approaches advocating variously for, for example: including participants as coresearchers (Frankena et al., 2019; Walmsley, 2001; Walmsley & The Central England People First History Project Team, 2014); engaging them as advisors or consultants with direct influence over the study's outcomes (Agboka, 2013; Kemmis, McTaggart, & Nixon, 2014; Spinuzzi, 2005); or adopting a more traditional approach with conventional researcher-participant roles (Holladay, 2017; Molloy, 2015; Uthappa, 2017). While participatory methodologies afford greater participant input, even more traditional research projects can be inclusive to the extent that the researcher remains sensitive to suggestions from participants and other stakeholders regarding the direction of the project, interpretation of findings, and representation of participant voices in data transcripts and publications (see Bivens, 2018; Carrion, 2020). Nevertheless, while the methodological pluralism that characterizes MHRR offers inclusive researchers a variety of methodological maps to choose from (see Scott & Melonçon, 2018), ethical tensions remain around topics such as responsibility, truth, power, relationships, and representation (McKinnon et al., 2016)—particularly in research involving people with mental health or mental disability diagnoses.

By virtue of its sensitivity to local contexts, MHRR offers an ideal disciplinary space to think through these tensions. Because inclusion is a rhetorical process, rhetorical field researchers, particularly those working in a feminist, decolonial, or interpretivist vein, are uniquely positioned to document what inclusive research looks and feels like in specific local contexts. I suggest that such researchers are also well

DOI: 10.4324/9781003144854-4

positioned to consider the manner in which the researcher's intersecting identities and prior experiences with/of inclusion shape their inclusive praxis. Specifically, I argue that by documenting the successes, failures, affordances, and constraints of their *inclusive research tactics*, MHR researchers can foster more inclusive understandings of rhetorical phenomena and forge more productive relationships with stakeholders. Inclusive research tactics, as I define them, are emergent methodological moves aimed at fostering greater inclusion in one's research practice. Such moves are tactical to the extent that they respond to novel problems and emergent situations that the researcher did not plan for. For example, Kristin Marie Bivens's (2018) advice to listen for "microwithdrawals of consent"—"the implied or partial halt of a person's willingness to participate in one or more aspects of the research process"—originated in a tactic she used in an unplanned encounter with a research participant (pp. 138–139). Carefully reading participants' body language for such withdrawals, as Bivens advises, includes participants by respecting their wishes, even when it results in losing them from the study.

In contrast to inclusive methods, inclusive research tactics originate not in established best practices, but in the researcher's unique inclusive orientation, or stance. To develop this notion further, I begin by defining the concept of inclusive research as it builds on existing literature and suggest how inclusive MHRR might exist alongside, and contribute to, more established traditions in social science fields, specifically by offering a rhetorical vision of inclusion as context-dependent. I then outline inclusion's rhetorical, localized dimensions by theorizing the relationship between the researcher's inclusive stance and their inclusion tactics, drawing on the work of Pierre Bourdieu (1991), Tanya Titchkosky (2011), Lisa Melonçon (2018), and Sara Ahmed (2006, 2012) to define inclusion as a kind of rhetorical disposition toward particular kinds of social actions. Next, I apply this framework to the case of the critical, ethical judgments I made as an able-bodied investigator on an IRB-approved study of an inclusive education program, exploring how my prior orientations toward inclusion were shaped by my work at a mental health nonprofit. Unconsciously applying these prior perspectives of inclusion to my research entailed certain affordances and constraints, helping me earn participants' trust while limiting my ability to engage in nuanced discussions of embodied difference with my participants, to productively analyze these differences, and to write about them. I conclude by offering a reflective tool researchers can use to better understand the affordances and limitations of their own habitual approaches to inclusion. By reflecting on the factors that make some inclusive tactics successful and others not, MHR researchers attempting inclusive interventions can expand their repertoire of effective inclusive strategies.

Inclusive Research Frameworks: Extant Approaches

Inclusion is one of the guiding ethical principles of the disability rights and consumer/survivor/ex-patient (c/s/x) movements. The iconic phrase "nothing about us without us" is frequently invoked in disability studies to make research more accountable to, and reflective of, disabled peoples' ways of knowing. This need is equally urgent in MHRR, given that much mental health research does not reflect the perspectives of people with mental health diagnoses (see McWade, Milton, & Beresford, 2015). MHRR thus faces a strong ethical imperative to craft research that includes the perspectives of participants and accounts for the researcher's role in describing and interpreting those perspectives.

In the social sciences, inclusive research encompasses a range of methodological approaches that, taken together, "reflect a particular turn towards democratization of the research process" (Nind, 2014, p. 1). Social scientists often use the term "inclusion" to refer specifically to the inclusion of people with intellectual/developmental disabilities (I/DDs)—or learning disabilities, as they are called in the UK, where much of this literature originates—in research about them.

Inclusive research in the learning disability field typically engages participants directly in research, from designing the study to publishing results (see Williams, 2011; Bigby, Frawley, & Ramcharan, 2014). Walmsley's collaboration with the Central England People's First (CEPF) History Project to research the history of the self-advocacy movement is an example of this approach (see Walmsley & The Central England People First History Project Team, 2014). Walmsley and the CEPF team determined the project's goals, designed its methodology, collected and analyzed the data, and cowrote the results together. Over the last 20 years, these practices have gradually spread to disciplines outside the learning disability field, including health research, as seen in Tessa Frankena et al.'s (2019) guidance statement to health researchers for recruiting researchers with disabilities and assigning researchers roles based on their strengths and interests.

In MHRR and adjacent fields, where interpretivist methodologies predominate, inclusion is invoked somewhat more loosely as a guiding value of social justice–oriented research and can be enacted in a variety of ways depending on the study context. Rhetoricians have long been interested in how scholars' values influence the outcomes of their research (see Jones, 2016; Scott & Melonçon, 2018). As Sullivan and Porter (1997) wrote,

> our research decisions are … guided by a vision of what constitutes a 'good' that we should be striving toward. It is this good, this political and ethical end, that we are trying to surface and critique when we talk about the importance of critical [reflexive] research practices.
>
> *(p. 8)*

As advocates, MHR researchers design their methodologies not only out of disciplinary means but also out of deeply felt commitments to some greater good, some benefit to society, or at minimum to the communities they work with/in and seek to address.

The spectrum of inclusive research frameworks available to MHR researchers thus spans from the 'merely' epistemologically inclusive, with the researcher acting as mediator of participant perspectives, to the more 'fully' inclusive, where participants are given direct access to the research process. My intention is not to advocate for any single approach, but to carve out space for a rhetorical theorization of inclusion as context-dependent. I advocate for a pluralistic perspective that recognizes various frameworks and practices as valid and generative. The key is for researchers to recognize how inclusive practices originate in local contexts and to appreciate inclusion as a felt, subjective, interpersonal (and hence, rhetorical) phenomenon. Understood rhetorically, inclusion can be thought of as something the researcher and their participant(s) cocreate, or coinvent, out of particular situations. This emphasis on the locally emergent justifies a more robust theorization of inclusive research tactics for MHRR.

Tactics and Orientations

Like many rhetoricians, I invoke the concept of tactics to describe in-the-moment responses to emergent rhetorical phenomena. Field-based research inevitably puts researchers in the position of having to respond quickly to what their participants say and do. Beyond participant interactions, the researcher must make ad hoc decisions about how to proceed with data collection and interpretation in the face of an ever-evolving research context. Tactics are not random; they are habitual responses to familiar situations. They are thus linked to Pierre Bourdieu's (1991) notion of habitus, the enduring dispositions of everyday action that influence how social agents act, behave, and perform. Habitus, Bourdieu explained, is not governed by official rules, but is acquired unconsciously. One's habitus reflects the social conditions in which they grow and live, persisting over time and across situations to produce perceptions and ways of being in fields other than originally intended (pp. 12–13).

Having an ethical commitment to an idea such as inclusion *orients* one's habitus toward a particular end, shaping their tactics. Adopting inclusion as an ethical orientation of MHRR thus requires attunement to one's habitual inclinations toward particular patterns of inclusive behaviors. In my case, growing up in a southern Christian household paradoxically meant learning deference and egalitarianism as core social dispositions, which influences how I enact inclusion for better or for worse. While habitus is not a totalizing force, understanding its influence is important for seeing the affordances and limitations of one's inclusive tactics.

Theorizing inclusive tactics is important for MHRR because it localizes inclusion, grounding it in the embodied knowledge of the researcher and their participants. The notion of orienting to inclusion recalls disability philosopher Tanya Titchkosky's (2011) theory of access as "a form of oriented social action" and "a way of relating to people and places" (p. 3). According to Titchkosky, access fundamentally involves a kind of direction, a pull toward relating to the world more openly and justly. Building on these ideas, and invoking Sara Ahmed's (2006) theory of orientation as concerning "how the bodily, the spatial, and the social are entangled" (qtd. in Melonçon, 2018, p. 39), Lisa Melonçon (2018) offered the idea of "orienting access" as a way of using practical everyday action to move toward greater access in institutional spaces such as the classroom (p. 46). This theorization of access as an orientation toward practical action lays the groundwork for a rhetorical understanding of inclusive research as an ethically oriented disposition whose goal is to erase barriers to equitable participation in the production of knowledge. Through studied reflection, inclusive researchers can come to understand the affordances and constraints of their predisposed inclusive tactics. In the following sections, I reflect on my own research process to illustrate the value of assessing one's own inclusive praxis for MHRR.

Study Background

Before describing my tactics, it is necessary to provide some background on my project, an IRB-approved study (IRB# 2017B0344) on the self-advocacy practices of rhetors with I/DDs.[1] The site for the project was an inclusive education program I refer to as STEP (Successful Transitions and Educational Empowerment). STEP offers a two- or four-year university certificate program providing coursework, internships, and social activities to students with qualified disability diagnoses. The purpose of my study was to better understand self-advocacy from a rhetorical perspective—an understanding I hoped would prove useful to my participants and to the larger disability community. For the first phase of the project, I interviewed five first-year STEP students about their self-advocacy experiences and analyzed several texts used to measure students' self-determination (see Kamperman, 2020a, 2020b). For the second phase, I interviewed a professional self-advocate affiliated with the program, Christine Brown,[2] who describes her work as speaking to elected officials on behalf of other people with disabilities to raise awareness for services such as STEP. I also conducted field observations of Brown advocating in meetings with elected officials and at a town hall (Kamperman, 2019).

My methodology, while not explicitly inclusive or participatory, mixed elements of grounded theory (Charmaz, 2008; Gasson, 2003; Tavory & Timmermans, 2014) and critical disability studies in an attempt to balance the participants' accounts of self-advocacy with my own theoretical perspectives/ explanations. Having no prior relationship with the STEP program, I relied on one of my committee members and longtime STEP supporter, Dr. T, to help me translate my research documents into language my participants and other stakeholders could appreciate. I also sought input from staff, participants, and friends and colleagues with disabilities on ethical questions related to recruitment, data collection, and representation.

Prior Experiences Performing Inclusion

When I began the project, my vision of how to make it inclusive was fuzzy at best. I did not realize how much my tactical interactions with participants and my methodological decision-making had been shaped by my nearly three years spent working at a mental health nonprofit. It is necessary to describe this work in order to flesh out how my inclusive research tactics emerged from prior experiences. This organization, a certified Clubhouse,[3] was a community-based program where membership was open to anyone with "a history of mental illness" (Clubhouse International, 2020). Clubhouses focus on community reintegration through meaningful work and relationships (to learn more about the Clubhouse model, see https://clubhouse-intl.org/about-us/mission-history/).

At its core, the Clubhouse is a nonclinical environment where people with psychiatric disabilities can gather safely to form a community around shared experiences, labor, and goals. The core values of the Clubhouse model are voluntarism, self-determination, and reintegration into community life, and members and staff work side-by-side at nearly every level of the organization. Because the model grew up alongside the disability rights and c/s/x movements of the 1960s and 1970s, it adheres firmly to the idea of self-determination and holds a healthy suspicion of psychiatric authority. The International Standards for Clubhouse Programs, which are ratified by the international Clubhouse community and reviewed every two years by a committee comprised of members and staff from accredited programs, stipulate that "all members have equal access to every Clubhouse opportunity with no differentiation based on diagnosis or level of functioning" and that "the work-ordered day must not include medication clinics, day treatment, or therapy programs within the Clubhouse" (Clubhouse International, 2016). Clubhouses are, for many, safe havens from the clinical gaze and places where members can develop relationships outside the patient-provider model of care.

With its emphasis on empowerment and its person-first approach to disability identity, the Clubhouse ingrained in me an inclusive habitus and an appreciation for difference, yet it did not prepare me to engage in nuanced discussions about many of the biological realities of mental disability diagnoses. The Clubhouse where I worked was fond of the saying that "Clubhouse members are known by their names, not their diagnoses," and did not prioritize hiring staff with clinical experience[4] (I myself had none). I rarely knew the specifics of a member's diagnosis beyond what they reported to me. Members were free to talk about their diagnoses to whomever they wished, but I rarely asked about them except during the intake process, leaving such discussions to more knowledgeable members and staff. This should not suggest that Clubhouses ignore difference; as Molloy (2015) observes, the Clubhouse where she conducted her research was a space where "the affordances of neurodiversity came through in ways that perhaps they would not have in more vertically arranged groups or more strictly clinical settings" (p. 142). The point is that the organization's policies created an environment where one's diagnosis was viewed as largely irrelevant to the Clubhouse work-ordered day.

It bears emphasizing that the stance toward disability/impairment I have characterized here is not the official position of Clubhouse International, nor that of the Clubhouse I worked for. In calling my stance the Clubhouse stance, I am using a bit of shorthand to denote the institutional origins of my felt orientation toward disability inclusion. This habitus developed semi-consciously, out of my interpretation of the norms, values, and practices of the Clubhouse setting.

To summarize, the Clubhouse stance toward inclusion is grounded in the following tenets:

- Self-determination
- Empowerment and a focus on strengths over vulnerabilities
- Emphasis on the idea of a universal personhood—person-first
- Reality of disability/impairment and cautious recognition of psychiatric authority
- Respect for privacy—diagnosis as a private matter
- Democratic decision-making

Inclusive Tactics that Yielded Affordances for the Research Process

This stance yielded many affordances in researching the STEP program. It helped me gain access to the research site, to engage potential participants, and to easily establish a rapport with those who eventually decided to participate. When I began my study, I instinctively attuned to the two sites' cultural similarities. Like the Clubhouse, the STEP program champions self-advocacy, self-determination, and empowerment as guiding principles. Students are supported in making independent choices about their programs of study, social activities, and accommodations and are coached on how to speak up for themselves in the classroom and in the workplace (see Grigal & Hart, 2010). These characteristics of the STEP program curriculum reflect the influence of the self-advocacy movement, whose mission is to help people with I/DD take greater control over their lives. Recognizing these features as similar to the Clubhouse, I resorted to my default inclusive orientation of treating the students as autonomous adults whose decision-making capacities I did not question. I saw this as necessary for gaining participants' trust and respect, without which the project's goals of truthfully documenting participants' voices/perspectives would not be possible.

My strategies for engaging with participants inclusively were to meet with them on their turf and communicate directly with the students whenever possible, rather than going through staff persons, instructors, or parents. Following the STEP program coordinator's advice, I made a recruitment pitch to the first-year STEP students during one of their classes and spent time getting to know them in the STEP tutoring center, where students hang out between classes. In these interactions, I instinctively did more listening than talking and watched carefully for body language and other emotional cues that might indicate discomfort (see Bivens, 2018; Ratcliffe, 2005). At the Clubhouse, we built an inclusive community through joking and informal talk. Though I was intensely nervous during my classroom presentation, where I was the supposed expert, I therefore felt at ease chatting with the students in the informal environment of the tutoring center. I quickly sensed that the students needed to test me before deciding to participate and that I would need to prove I was trustworthy by showing that we had shared interests (sports, videogames, etc.) and that I had a sense of humor. Another Clubhouse value steering my interactions with participants was that of egalitarian, shoulder-to-shoulder work. Though I did not seriously consider enlisting participants as coinvestigators due to time and funding constraints, I tried to make myself useful to the STEP community. This was accomplished primarily through small, spontaneous gestures, such as offering to share my field notes with self-advocate Christine Brown and her team, taking minutes during an important meeting, and setting up tables and chairs before a townhall. I instinctively positioned myself as ready to help out and eager to learn, as I had done at the Clubhouse. These gestures convinced Christine of my sincerity and helped create a more egalitarian researcher-participant relationship.

Bringing this egalitarian ethos to my interviews yielded unexpected methodological affordances. Because Clubhouses place such importance on ordinary conversation as a space where, in Margaret Price's (2011) words, "power is exchanged" (p. 60), I instinctively gravitated toward a less formal, semi-structured interview style. The principles of self-advocacy and self-determination foreground talk as a space where one "tak[es] control of one's life" (Williams, 2011, p. 3). I thus let participants go on in their interviews, even when it led us astray from my original list of questions. To create the feeling of a conversation, I interjected frequently to reflect back my understanding of participants' perspectives and clarify/contour their remarks. While planning the project, Dr. T and I agreed that if a participant did not know the term self-advocacy, I should define it as "standing up for myself" (e.g., "Tell me about a time you stood up for yourself") or simply redirect the conversation toward an adjacent concept, such as disclosure of the student's goals ("Tell me about how you accomplish your goals"). It wasn't until well into data analysis that I fully grasped the epistemological implications of this open-ended, conversational approach. By participating actively in the interview process, I became a more active cocreator of the rhetorical acts I was seeking to analyze and understand. While hardly problematic or surprising from a rhetorical viewpoint (see Clarke, 2005), this forced me to productively revise some of my claims, in particular the assertion that my project was straightforwardly about documenting and amplifying marginalized voices. Introducing concepts such as "stand up for myself" into the conversation reified the hegemonic understandings of self-advocacy I was attempting to critique—a point brought to my attention by an editor who asked me to clarify my methodological position and situate myself more clearly in the research narrative as a coproducer of hegemonic self-advocacy discourse (Kamperman, 2020a). While a different inclusive tactic in this case—perhaps one oriented toward letting participants talk uninterrupted rather than explaining concepts— might have yielded a more straightforward record of participants' perceptions of self-advocacy, I believe my approach yielded a no less valuable dialectical, coconstructivist account of hegemonic self-advocacy discourse.

Inclusive Tactics that Yielded Methodological Limitations

While in many respects my habituated inclusive tactics contributed to my project's goals of including the voices of people with I/DD in rhetorical research, in some cases they impeded these efforts. This section discusses two tactics that yielded limitations for the project: my failure to appreciate the rhetorical complexity of the recruitment encounter, and my inclination to avoid discussions of bodily difference. This second tactic hampered my ability to gather useful data and led to a normative account of participants' self-advocacy practices. It also led to difficulties in selecting appropriate terminology to describe participants' identity/embodiment. I describe how some alternative inclusive tactics would have been beneficial in these areas.

My unexamined instinct to view the students, all of whom were 18 or older, as fully capable of deciding for themselves whether they wished to participate in the study underestimated the rhetorical complexity of research involving cognitive disability, leading to two missteps. First, I neglected the role parents and legal guardians might play in helping some students decide whether or not to participate. While I advised every student to discuss their decision with their parents, I did not attempt to engage the parents directly; I felt that doing so might signify a lack of confidence in the students' own decision-making skills. Second, I tended not to follow up with students who signaled any hesitancy about participating. My interactions with one student whom I'll refer to as Trey exhibit the consequences of this tactic. After striking up a conversation with Trey in the tutoring center, I took out a pen and began jotting down his contact information, to which he remarked: "So you take notes on what we say and stuff?" I thought I detected in his question a note of suspicion, or disappointment that our casual conversation had seemingly turned into an unauthorized field observation. When Trey later declined to participate in the study, saying he was too busy that fall but that he might be able to in the spring, I thought back to our initial interaction and wondered if his offer of a follow-up was simply him being polite. I ended up not following up with him, feeling that it would have been pushy. I realize now that this tactical interpretation of Trey's behavior was grounded in an assumption that he, like I, viewed research as a power-laden transaction with significant potential for harm. My concern was not necessarily misplaced; in research involving people with diagnoses of cognitive and IDs, or who experience temporary or "ephemeral" intellectual disablement due to trauma, medication side effects, or other factors, it is advisable for researchers to be highly attuned to participants' embodied language throughout the study, including "microwithdrawals of consent" (Bivens, 2018, pp. 138–139). However, as I became familiar with the culture of the STEP program, I realized that STEP students routinely participate in research. I recognize now that Trey's remark about my notetaking could have come from a place of curiosity rather than a place of suspicion. By relying on a habitual stance to treat all participants as fully self-aware and autonomous—as "consenting adults" with an inherent distrust of researchers—I perhaps mistakenly assumed that participants would make up their minds fairly quickly about me and my project. This episode shows how, in the kairotic space (Price, 2011) of the recruitment encounter, enacting inclusion might necessitate giving potential participants multiple ways *into* the study as well as multiple ways out (Bivens), especially in studies involving participants who may have difficulty processing information the first time they receive it. In ethnographic research involving people with cognitive disabilities, it may be appropriate in certain cases to remind potential participants about one's project and invite them to participate more than once, tactics that in other settings might seem overly persistent. An alternative inclusive tactic in this situation would have been to tactfully follow up with Trey in the spring to ask if he'd given any more thought to the project.

Another tactic that proved consequential was my instinct not to ask participants about their disabilities. While my Clubhouse experience habituated me to neurodiversity, it did not prepare me to initiate frank discussions about the reality of impairment, or what disability studies scholar Tobin Siebers (2008) referred to as complex embodiment. As a nondisabled person, I had not learned how to frame questions about participants' disabilities in a way that felt inclusive (nonothering). Moreover, legally, STEP students have a right to keep medical information confidential, according to the Family Educational Rights and Privacy Act (FERPA) and Health Insurance Portability and Accountability Act (HIPAA). Given the stigma attached to mental disability, STEP staff counsel students to exercise careful judgment when deciding whether to disclose (see Freedman, Eisenman, Grigal, & Hart, 2017, p. 294). The research's institutional context thus made it fairly easy to avoid initiating conversations about participants' disabilities. This led me to rest on the comfortable, if erroneous assumption that inclusion could be achieved by focusing on similarities rather than differences.

This assumption led to a lack of imagination concerning participants' access needs. In particular, I failed to anticipate that some participants might have nonnormative ways of communicating. To counteract such assumptions, Stephanie Kerschbaum and Margaret Price (2017) advised centering disability in the interview process: "Centering disability … means posing the question: If we *assume* that disability is part of the qualitative-interview situation, how does that unsettle commonplace assumptions about qualitative interviewing" (p. 98)? Accordingly, my decision not to video-record my interviews—a choice made early in my project out of concern that participants who preferred to remain anonymous might be made uncomfortable by the presence of a camera—was inclusive in intent, but not in effect. I assumed that audio recording my interviews would suffice to capture participants' rhetoric, an assumption that proved wrong in the case of a participant with a speech impairment whom I'll refer to as Simon. Because Simon's speech is difficult for most interlocutors (myself included) to understand, he augments his speech with hand gestures, as well as a tapping technique and (occasionally) a smartphone app that helps him to control the tempo of his speech. Without a camera, I was unable to fully capture how Simon communicates. It wasn't just Simon's communication that was flattened by the lack of video; I too access face-to-face interaction aurally and visually, through modalities such as gesture and facial expression, as do the other students I interviewed. Thus, in my attempts to enact inclusion by using recording techniques I perceived as less threatening to participants' privacy, I paradoxically precluded access to data that could have provided a richer impression of self-advocacy's embodied, interactive dimensions. While an IRB amendment to incorporate video recording into the methods likely would have been approved, I had run out of time to collect any new data by the time this dilemma surfaced. A more effective inclusive tactic would have been to state in my IRB protocol that participants could have the option of a video- or audio recorded interview.

Further, while the intent behind my choice of a grounded theory methodology was inclusive, this too yielded limitations. Grounded theory strives to promote reflexivity and accountability through practices such as reflexive memoing and iterative coding. These practices, while promoting sensitivity to researcher bias, also privilege patterns and similarities between participants at the expense of difference. Committing to grounded theory coding techniques (see Gasson, 2003) resulted in Simon's transcript in particular becoming an analytical outlier. Because so much of my interview with Simon was focused on our efforts to communicate—as opposed to Simon's thoughts on self-advocacy—the codes I used to describe Simon's rhetorical performances tended to focus on meta-communication: for example, "Asking to repeat" (23x), "Checking understanding" (9x), "Recognizing misunderstanding and voluntarily repeating" (4x), "Breaking response into parts to increase understanding" (3x),

"Collaboratively breaking down response" (2x), and "Spelling out words to help with understanding" (1x). By contrast, the codes I generated for the other transcripts tended to be more thematic ("Talking about asking for help," "Identifying strengths and weaknesses," "Using support network," etc.). While some grounded theorists encourage researchers to explore such outliers, I gradually stopped coding the other transcripts' meta-communicative elements as I became increasingly engrossed in their thematic content. Thus, one consequence of adopting a coding methodology that was intended to filter out my biases was that it steered me toward a normative account of student self-advocacy practices that was not entirely sensitive to bodily difference. A potentially better inclusive tactic in this instance would have been to center difference/disability in my decisions about which data to include in my analysis rather than treating Simon's transcript as an outlier.

Inclusive Tactics with Mixed Effects

The ethical consequences of the final tactic I describe—my decision to use varied terminology in my descriptions of participants—were more ambiguous. As I began writing up my results, I was quickly confronted with difficult choices about how to represent my participants' identities. Another consequence of my hesitancy to ask participants about their disabilities was that I did not know how the majority of my participants identified. At the time, I did not perceive this to be a major issue, since every participant but Christine Brown chose to remain anonymous. Even had I known this information, I still would be faced with the representational dilemma of having to use blanket terms to describe people with diverse abilities and identities. I thus turned to other scholarship for guidance. While many in the inclusive education field refer to participants using person-first language (PFL), e.g., "people with I/DD," not all scholars and activists agree with this approach (see Brown, 2011). These conflicts are especially pronounced in the Mad, I/DD, autistic, and self-advocacy communities, where many reject diagnostic labels, and disability identity altogether, as oppressive, while others choose to embrace disability (for a nuanced discussion, see Price, 2011, pp. 9–20). The following examples from my own research reflect the diversity of my participants' orientations toward disability:

- Self-advocate Christine Brown advocated for PFL when referring to people with I/DD. Her choice to be identified "as a person with a disability who advocates on behalf of others with disabilities" bespeaks her view that she, and those she represents, are not defined by their disabilities.
- Gregg, a STEP student, seemed at ease talking about his diagnoses and how his disabilities affect his learning and behavior, but did not share how he identifies.
- Marc, on the other hand, also a student, talked openly about trying to overcome his disabilities:

I grew out of it because I don't see myself … bein shy anymore … all of my, you know, learning disabilities, like … I've faced a lot of em and I know what I have and what I don't have and like, what I can do and what I cannot do … I mean reading's still a huge … problem, and writing, and y'know math … but y'know … I'm fighting it … that's all I can do from autism and ADHD, ya just gotta fight it.

Even though philosophically I view assertions of disability-first identity as important for creating a society more tolerant of vulnerability, interdependence, and difference, as an able-bodied, cisgender man, I felt that it was not my place to challenge my participants' understandings of/orientations to disability, and that doing so would violate the inclusive spirit of the project. Thus, when it came time to write up my results, I attempted to split the difference among these various orientations by using the cumbersome phrase "people who identify as or are identified as having an intellectual/developmental disability." For brevity's sake, elsewhere in the write-up I defaulted to PFL ("people with I/DD"). I occasionally used disability-first language, but never in reference to Brown, and I tended to avoid reference to specific diagnostic categories as I have done throughout this essay. My use of broad diagnostic categories such as I/DD and, in some instances, "mental disability" was intended to be broadly inclusive, yet it had the disadvantage of lacking the specificity necessary to express nuanced differences between participants' embodiments. This issue was brought to my attention during my dissertation defense by Dr. T, who expressed concern that my terminology was overly ambiguous and pushed me to clarify what I meant by "I/DD" more clearly. Dr. T's perspective as a parent of someone with disabilities forced me to confront the limitations of a broad approach to disability representation: by habitually ignoring the medical meanings of particular terms, however fraught, I risked omitting relevant information about my participants that would shed light on their rhetorical performances. MHR researchers inevitably face representational dilemmas such as these. Acknowledging how one's representational tactics are formed, while not a solution to the important philosophical questions underlying these debates, at minimum situates one's research vis-à-vis local practices and customs.

Conclusion

A rhetorical understanding of inclusion as both context-dependent and grounded in the researcher's habitus can reveal the affordances and limitations of a plurality of approaches to inclusive research. As my case hopefully demonstrates, how one performs inclusive research on a tactical level can matter for knowledge. Working at a Clubhouse conditioned me to orient toward disability as a private matter, to focus on participants' strengths and competencies rather than vulnerabilities, to view participants as fully autonomous, to position myself as a nonexpert, and to try to use the most inclusive language possible. This stance had certain affordances and limitations which became apparent to me upon reflection. While one's habitual approach to enacting inclusion might not be actively harmful, it is worth considering how inclusive tactics developed in one context might limit inclusion in another. I thus conclude this chapter by describing an iterative reflective process researchers can use to similarly take stock of their own inclusive habits and tactics. While I did not use this process in my own research, it does grow out of my project. My hope is that others can use it to reflect more deeply on their inclusive habitus and adjust their tactics as necessary.

The first step in the process is simply to reflect on one's previous experiences of inclusion. These reflections need not be limited to research; they could include examples from teaching, service, or committee work. Try to recall specific inclusive actions and the language used to describe those actions. The more details you are able to remember, the better. For each experience, name the settings, actors, and actions whereby inclusion was performed. Flesh out the context of these inclusive acts by listing the cultural/discursive, material/economic, and social/political features of the settings or activity systems in which they occurred.[5] Doing so will help keep your emergent understanding of inclusion localized and grounded.

The second step is to articulate a definition of inclusion based on these prior experiences. This definition can be a sentence or two or a bulleted list like the one I used above to enumerate the Clubhouse's inclusive tenets. It may be helpful at this stage to articulate what you envision inclusion looking like at each stage of the research process: planning, recruitment, data collection, data analysis, publication, and so on. Return to this definition periodically and update it as needed.

Once you have generated a working definition of inclusion and reflected on its connection to prior experiences, the third step is to construct a table comparing prior and emerging contexts of inclusion (see Table 2.1 for an example). The goal of this step is to consider how inclusion is normally understood and enacted at the research site compared to other settings. You can use the descriptive categories cultural/discursive, material/economic, and social/political to organize salient features of inclusion at the sites you are comparing. Documenting inclusion's material/economic features promotes awareness of how even within a single site, the norms around inclusion can shift room-to-room (for example, the STEP tutoring center was, informally, a student space; students thus had more agency there compared to, say, the classroom). Updating this table throughout the project can help you identify tactics that may be ill-adapted to the research context. In my case, visualizing contrasting features of the Clubhouse and the STEP program could have helped me recognize that compared to Clubhouse members, it is normal for STEP students to receive support in making decisions about their participation in the program.

In addition to these steps, like Melissa Carrion (2020), I advocate that reflexive strategies such as memoing be used early in the research process to attune

TABLE 2.1 Comparison of Prior and Emerging Contexts of Inclusion

	(A) Norms Around Inclusion	
(B) Features of Inclusion	Prior Context (Clubhouse)	Emerging Context (STEP Program)
Cultural-discursive	Person-first language; service users referred to as "members," not clients; cultural connection to c/s/x movement	Person-first language; emphasis on self-advocacy and self-determination
Material-economic	All members have access to every part of the Clubhouse; work is voluntary and unpaid; Clubhouse members do not pay for services; Clubhouse facilities are ADA accessible	STEP students have access to all campus spaces and activities, including spaces that "belong" to them (e.g., the tutoring center); STEP students pay tuition to attend, usually with financial aid; program facilities are ADA accessible
Social-political	Members make decisions independently and work shoulder-to-shoulder with staff; members are empowered to participate in all group decisions and have representation on Board of Directors; nonhierarchical social relationships; members express agency through joking with staff	STEP students attend classes with the general student population and participate in campus social activities; STEP students are supported in making decisions about courses, accommodations, social activities, and internships in annual Person-Centered Planning meetings, which they lead; parents are usually present for these meetings; students do not have direct ownership over the curriculum; students express agency through joking with staff

the researcher to their unique stances/orientations. Because the individual values shaping one's choice and implementation of a particular methodology are not always apparent, reflexivity is essential to any qualitative researcher's process. Practices such as journaling and theoretical memoing can attune the researcher to their evolving perspective and hedge against reductive explanations of phenomena (Charmaz, 2008, p. 166). Finally, researchers should make their inclusive strategies and tactics explicit in their study narratives and clarify the affordances and limitations of their approach. If one's inclusive orientation offers a matrix of possibilities for enacting inclusive research, then surfacing these tactics can help reveal inclusion's rhetorical nuances. This rhetorical take on inclusion can complement more established approaches to inclusive research in the social sciences, making research interventions in MHR more inclusive and, one hopes, just.

Notes

1 In centering the concept of disability, I am making a meaningful interpretive move, or agential cut (Barad, 2003, 2007), that many members of the Mad and c/s/x movements would likely find ontologically objectionable. While acknowledging I/DD's material-discursive distinctiveness from forms of psychiatric disability such as depression, schizophrenia, and bipolar, in the spirit of inclusion, I attempt to bring the categories together under the umbrella term "mental disability," following the example of Margaret Price (2011) in her book *Mad at School*. This move speaks to a recognition that people who exhibit mental differences (neurodivergence), whether emotional, perceptual, or cognitive in nature, often experience similar oppressions, and focuses attention on how disability becomes manifest in routinized, institutional environments.
2 Christine Brown has given me permission to use her real name.
3 Cathryn Molloy's (2015) article for *Rhetoric Society Quarterly*, "Recuperative Ethos and Agile Epistemologies: Toward a Vernacular Engagement with Mental Illness Ontologies," is based on research done at a Clubhouse. She provides a detailed look at the organization's culture, in particular how the Clubhouse functions as an environment where members can reestablish ethos through everyday vernacular performances.
4 It is worth noting that not all Clubhouses operate this way.
5 I borrow these categories from *The Action Research Planner* by Stephen Kemmis, Robin McTaggart, and Rhonda Nixon (2014), who use them to describe the contextual dimensions of social practices.

References

Agboka, Godwin Y. (2013). Participatory localization: A social justice approach to navigating unenfranchised/disenfranchised cultural sites. *Technical Communication Quarterly, 22*(1), 28–49.

Ahmed, Sara. (2006). *Queer phenomenology: Orientations, objects, others.* Duke University Press.

Ahmed, Sara. (2012). *On being included: Racism and diversity in institutional life.* Duke University Press.

Barad, Karen. (2003). Posthumanist performativity: Toward an understanding of how matter comes to matter. *Signs: Journal of Women in Culture and Society, 28*(3), 801–831.

Barad, Karen. (2007). *Meeting the universe halfway: Quantum physics and the entanglement of matter and meaning.* Duke University Press.

Bigby, Christine, Frawley, Patsie and Ramcharan, Paul. (2014). Conceptualizing inclusive research with people with intellectual disability. *Journal of Applied Research in Intellect Disabilities, 27*(1), 3–12. https://doi.org/10.1111/jar.12083

Bivens, Kristin M. (2018). Rhetorically listening for microwithdrawals of consent in research practice. In Lisa Meloncon & J. Blake Scott (Eds.), *Methodologies for the rhetoric of health & medicine* (pp. 138–56). Routledge.

Bourdieu, Pierre. (1991). *Language and symbolic power.* Harvard University Press.

Brown, Lydia. (2011, November 30). *Person-first language: Why it matters (the significance of semantics).* The Thinking Person's Guide to Autism. http://www.thinkingautismguide.com/2011/11/person-first-language-why-it-matters.html/

Carrion, Melissa. (2020). Negotiating the ethics of representation in RHM research. *Rhetoric of Health & Medicine, 3*(4), 437–448. doi:10.5744/rhm.2020.4005

Charmaz, Kathy. (2008). Grounded theory as emergent method. In Sharlene N. Hesse-Biber & Patricia Leavy (Eds.), *Handbook of Emergent Methods* (pp. 155–170). Guilford Press.

Clarke, Adele E. (2005). *Situational analysis.* SAGE Publications, Inc.

Clubhouse International. (2016). *International standards for clubhouse programs.* Retrieved January 7, 2021 from https://www.clubhouse-intl.org/documents/standards_2016_eng.pdf

Clubhouse International. (2020). Retrieved January 7, 2021 from https://clubhouse-intl.org/.

Frankena, Tessa K., Naaldenberg, Jenneken, Cardol, Mieke, Garcia Iriarte, Edurne, Buchner, Tobias, Brooker, Katie, Embregts, Petri, Joosa, Esther, Crowther, Felicity, Fudge Schormans, Ann, Schippers, Alice, Walmsley, Jan, O'Brien, Patricia, Linehan, Christine, Northway, Ruth, van Schrojenstein Lantman-de Valk, Henry, and Leusink, Geraline. (2019). A consensus statement on how to conduct inclusive health research. *Journal of Intellectual Disability Research, 63*(1), 1–11. https://doi.org/10.1111/jir.12486.

Freedman, Brian, Eisenman, Laura T., Grigal, Meg, & Hart, Debra. (2017). Intellectual disability in the university: Expanding the conversation about diversity and disclosure. In Stephanie L. Kerschbaum, Laura T. Eisenman, & James M. Jones (Eds.), *Negotiating disability: Disclosure and higher education* (pp. 291–310). University of Michigan Press.

Gasson, Susan. (2003). Rigor in grounded theory research: An interpretive perspective on generating theory from qualitative field studies. In Michael E. Whitman & Amy B. Woszczyynski (Eds.), *The handbook of information systems research* (pp. 79–102). Idea Group Publishing.

Grigal, Meg, & Hart, Debra. (2010). *Think college!: Postsecondary education options for students with intellectual disabilities.* Paul H. Brookes Publishing Company.

Holladay, Drew. (2017). Classified conversations: Psychiatry and tactical technical communication in online spaces. *Technical Communication Quarterly, 26*(1), 8–24.

Jones, Natasha N. (2016). The technical communicator as advocate: Integrating a social justice approach in technical communication. *Journal of Technical Writing and Communication, 46*(3), 342–361.

Kamperman, Sean A. (2019). *Intellectual/developmental disability, rhetoric, and self-advocacy: A case study.* (Electronic Thesis or Dissertation). Retrieved from https://etd.ohiolink.edu/

Kamperman, Sean A. (2020a). Academic ableism and students with intellectual/developmental disabilities: Rethinking self-advocacy as an anti-ableist practice. *Critical Education, (11)*17. https://doi.org/10.14288/ce.v11i17.186501

Kamperman, Sean A. (2020b). Recognizing the *métis* of learners with intellectual/developmental disabilities in college composition. (Roundtable). *Disability Studies Quarterly, 40*(1). https://doi.org/10.18061/dsq.v40i1.7223

Kemmis, Stephen, McTaggart, Robbin, & Nixon, Rhonda. (2014). *The action research planner: Doing critical participatory action research.* Springer Science & Business Media.

Kerschbaum, Stephanie L., & Price, Margaret. (2017). Centering disability in qualitative interviewing. *Research in the Teaching of English, 52*(1), 98–107.

McKinnon, Sara L., Johnson, Jenell, Asen, Robert, Chavez, Karma R., & Howard, Robert G. (2016). Rhetoric and ethics revisited: What happens when rhetorical scholars go into the field. *Cultural Studies Critical Methodologies, 16*(6), 560–570. doi:10.1177/1532708616659080

McWade, Brigit, Milton, Damian, & Beresford, Peter. (2015). Mad studies and neuro-diversity: A dialogue, *Disability & Society, 30*(2), 305–309, doi:10.1080/09687599.2 014.1000512

Melonçon, Lisa. (2018). Orienting access in our business and professional communication classrooms. *Business and Professional Communication Quarterly, 81*(1), 34. doi:10.1177/2329490617739885

Molloy, Cathryn. (2015). Recuperative ethos and agile epistemologies: Toward a vernacular engagement with mental illness ontologies. *Rhetoric Society Quarterly, 45*(2), 138–163. doi:10.1080/02773945.2015.1010125

Nind, Melanie. (2014). *What is inclusive research?* Bloomsbury Academic. doi:10.5040/9781849668149

Price, Margaret. (2011). *Mad at school: Rhetorics of mental disability and academic life.* University of Michigan Press.

Ratcliffe, Krista. (2005). *Rhetorical listening: Identification, gender, whiteness.* Southern Illinois University Press.

Scott, J. Blake, & Melonçon, Lisa. (2018). Manifesting methodologies for the rhetoric of health & medicine. In Lisa Melonçon & J. Blake Scott (Eds.), *Methodologies for the rhetoric of health & medicine* (pp. 1–23). Routledge.

Siebers, Tobin. (2008). *Disability theory.* University of Michigan Press.

Spinuzzi, Clay. (2005). The methodology of participatory design. *Technical Communication, 52*(2), 163–174.

Sullivan, Patricia, & Porter, James. (1997). *Opening spaces: Writing technologies and critical research practices.* Ablex.

Tavory, Iddo, & Timmermans, Stephan. (2014). *Abductive analysis: Theorizing qualitative research.* University of Chicago Press.

Titchkosky, Tanya. (2011). *The question of access: Disability, space, meaning.* University of Toronto Press.

Uthappa, N. Renuka. (2017). Moving closer: Speakers with mental disabilities, deep disclosure, and agency through vulnerability. *Rhetoric Review, 36*(2), 164–175.

Walmsley, Jan. (2001). Normalisation, emancipatory research and inclusive research in learning disability. *Disability & Society, 16*(2), 187–205.

Walmsley, Jan, & The Central England People First History Project Team. (2014). Telling the history of self-advocacy: A challenge for inclusive research. *Journal of Applied Research in Intellectual Disabilities, 27*(1), 34–43. https://doi.org/10.1111/jar.12086

Williams, Val. (2011). *Disability and discourse: Analysing inclusive conversation with people with intellectual disabilities.* Wiley-Blackwell.

3

CULTURE-CENTERED APPROACHES TO RHETORICAL RESEARCH

Considering Domestic Violence as a Site for Intersectional Interventions

Lisa DeTora and Tomeka Robinson

Why Domestic Violence?

Domestic violence is associated with stressful circumstances and situations that force families into closer quarters than usual, creating mental and emotional tensions that can result in violent outbursts (Abramson, 2020). In the early months of the COVID-19 pandemic, for instance, media discussions of domestic violence linked an uptick in cases to mental health problems, such as depression, and to stay-at-home orders (Stone, 2020; Taub, 2020). An obstacle to intervening in such violence is both rhetorical and seemingly contradictory: an absence of reports may signal worse danger than an increase in complaints (Stone, 2020). The rhetorical problems of domestic violence do not end with a tension between speaking and not speaking. Quotations from the United Nations, urging attention to "women's safety" (Taub, 2020) in this context reveal that many discussions of domestic violence carry specific assumptions about gender and family relationships, signaling the possibility for additional discursive elisions. If "domestic violence" codes as "male violence against female sexual partners," then many sufferers, including children and the elderly, become invisible. A focus on heteronormative couplings means that people living in so-called nontraditional family patterns may face additional barriers to obtaining needed support.

The more narrowly any site of public health intervention is defined, the more susceptible already marginalized people are to harm. Culture-centered approaches have the potential to illuminate and overcome these barriers and afford researchers new methodological approaches to their work. However, merely appending a culture-centered approach to the current situation misses important opportunities for rhetorical intervention. Below, we present a

DOI: 10.4324/9781003144854-5

heuristic for culture-centered inquiry and situate it relative to domestic violence research, its rhetorics, and its history to identify possible sites for scholarly intervention. Our suggestions integrate culture-centered, theoretical, and narrative methods gleaned from health communications, rhetoric, and bioethics to produce a more nuanced and complex approach to domestic violence and other complicated and multifaceted health situations.

Culture-Centered Approaches as Intersectional Inquiry

Our call for more culture-centered approaches to domestic violence rhetorics parallels those of sociologist Melvina Sumter (2006) and legal expert Kimberlé Crenshaw (1991) for interventions into domestic violence that address multicultural contexts and elements of race, class, and gender that, as suggested by Patricia Collins and others (1998, 2000; Andersen & Collins, 2004; See also Appleby, Colon, & Hamilton, 2007), are necessary to understand all human experience. That the original calls were made so long ago signals an ongoing need to address persistent social and cultural inequities. Intersectionality is a conceptual framework and methodology for practice and research founded in Black Feminism as a way to account for various facets of identity in concrete, material, positional ways (Crenshaw, 1991; Lockhart & Danis, 2010). Intersectionality accounts for how race, ethnicity, class, gender, sex, sexual orientation, and/or sexual identity impact access to power and privilege as well as how this access influences personal and social perceptions and beliefs (Crenshaw, 1991). Intersectionality allows for a wider critical frame compared with many other approaches to identity and can be used to explore norms and power in relation to a broad range of identities in health communication (Spieldenner, Robinson, & Woodruffe, 2019). Intersectional theory also shifts the blame for inequities from individuals to social structures in order to highlight the origins of social problems. While intersectional theory has not yet, to our knowledge, been used to address domestic violence in health communication or rhetorical scholarship, we see a lot of promise for this approach.

Within the context of domestic violence, as sociologist Natalie Sokoloff (2008) explained, an intersectional framework acknowledges that people have multiple, layered identities that interact and contribute to their unique experiences of oppression, marginalization, and violence. Crenshaw (1991) noted that intersectionality must be used to understand the experiences of women of color subject to violence at home as they interact with police and the courts. Crenshaw's "From Private Violence to Mass Incarceration: Thinking Intersectionally about Women, Race, and Social Control" (2012) also described the double-binds faced by women of color and their partners in a society that *de facto* marginalizes and excludes persons of color. Clearly, in a legal system that routinely seeks to imprison Black people, the stakes of reporting domestic violence might alter significantly. And existing scholarship shows that domestic violence is only one situation in which race, class, and ethnicity can play out in negative ways for already marginalized people (Appleby, Colon, & Hamilton, 2007; Collins, 1998, 2000). While intersectionality allows us to understand layered identities, it doesn't account for how rhetorical or communication interventions can and should work. A culture-centered approach to health communication, however, can consider how structure, culture, and agency play out in the specific circumstances faced by particular persons, and may allow individuals within the system to co-construct interventions that are responsive and appropriate.

The Need for Culture-Centered Approaches to Mental Health Rhetoric Research

As rhetors and scholars, we must identify ways to better incorporate intersectionality and culture-centered approaches into our work. Without a deeper, multilayered understanding, we fail our communities and may uphold ideologies that further marginalize the vulnerable. Culture-centered approaches to health communication grow out of basic ethical questions about which people have access to needed resources and care. Both individual and social biases influence the degree to which cultural information about human subjects, patients, and caregivers is included or excluded from discursive contexts like healthcare decision-making or rhetorical study. Mohan Dutta (2007, 2008, 2018), an expert in examining marginalization and poverty as social issues, developed a culture-centered approach to health communication. Dutta seeks to address criticisms of traditional health models that elide certain voices by recognizing the narratives that emerge through conversations with members of marginalized communities. In a culture-centered approach to communication, structure focuses on the aspects of social organization that simultaneously constrain and enable participants to participate in health-related behaviors. Culture is illustrated by the day-to-day practices of members within a community: within a health context, interpretation of health, wellness, and illness are socially constructed. Agency is the capacity of people to enact their choices and to participate actively in negotiating the structures in which they live. Structure, culture, and agency are each subject to rhetorical pressures based on prior assumptions about normative family life that go beyond the "family systems" approaches to domestic violence suggested in the 1980s (Gelles & Maynard, 1987).

Traditionally, rhetorical approaches to mental (and other) health frameworks, as J. Fred Reynolds (2018) noted, have manifested an individual-level focus as well as cognitive, decontextualized, and control biases. Dutta's culture-centered approach, in contrast, seeks to build spaces for meaningful discourse to interrogate, theorize, and formulate ways to critically probe the power structures built into the production of knowledge within the fields of medicine and public health. Scholars utilizing a culture-centered approach to health communication should look critically at the scientific facts embedded in health interventions and understand the complex ways that structure, culture, and agency interact within these exchanges.

Culture reflects the shared values, practices, and meanings that are negotiated within communities. It is simultaneously static and dynamic, in that it passes on values within the community, while also creating opportunities for transforming those values over time. Structure focuses on the communicative resources, rules, and assumptions within a community. These structures are constituted within larger social, political, and economic structures and are directly connected to power within social systems. Agency is the enactment of everyday choices by community members who are both enabled and constrained by the structures in place. Culture, structure, and agency communicatively interact with each other, and the predominate emphasis is to creative spaces where those who are in marginalized positions can co-create their theoretical frameworks and develop solutions. As Dutta (2018) explained,

> whereas agency is communicatively expressed, the process of communication draws upon cultural meanings, and is located in relationship to structures. Co-creating legitimate spaces for recognition and representation of hitherto erased meanings offer an entry point to the development of culturally grounded solutions…the solutions proposed are often material in the form of the development of infrastructures and services, and in other instances, are discursive, in the form of creation of communication campaigns and advocacy tools, grounded in community voices.
>
> *(p. 241)*

The framework of the culture-centered approach is driven toward theory-building and highlighting solutions that emerge from within communities (Dutta, 2007). Co-creation here is a critical term that allows space for rhetorical articulations to encompass more than one unified position, allowing for the development of authentically new perspectives.

By building on Dutta's culture-centered approach, rhetors and scholars can consider multiple elements that inform the situation of domestic violence more effectively. Collecting and considering information about culture, resources, social structures, and personal agency is an important way to interrogate sites of power and marginalization—particularly in ways that are responsive to intersectional complexities. Dominant social actors may maintain their control over the social system through economic access, which might become obscured when dealing with individual, snapshot views of domestic violence. When considering mental health and domestic violence constructions, power is maintained through the naming process of what is considered domestic violence and who has the power in deciding how and when to intervene. In situations like shelter-in-place orders, these questions and their answers might assist rhetorical analysis that resists cultural stories that normalize a white, heteronormative family structure while eliding other household and social arrangements.

A Culture-Centered Intervention Framework for Mental Health Rhetoric Research

If we identify elements of social structures, culture, and agency that impact individuals and rhetorical situations, it becomes more feasible to design and engage in effective rhetorical intervention, particularly in contexts like domestic violence that require attention to multiple facts of experience for different people within an already complex social situation. To this end, we developed a heuristic that can be used to collect information that would be needed to engage in effective rhetorical research in such settings. We sought to identify critical elements of social structures, culture, and personal agency that might impact how domestic violence is discussed as a mental health problem with the potential for causing public health impact, following from the remarks with which we opened this paper.

In Table 3.1, we take the example of an undocumented immigrant domestic worker, considering that domestic violence discourses during public health emergencies like COVID-19 may be informed by certain presumptions about bourgeois heteronormativity. In walking through the elements of a culture-centered approach, it seems clear that essential information is lacking and complex cultural identities are not adequately included in some of the dominant discourses of domestic violence we cited earlier. For example, an undocumented immigrant domestic worker who is a non-English speaker occupies an intersectional identity that places them in a more vulnerable position for abuse and death from COVID-19 even before they might experience (or witness) physical or sexual assault at home. This position also changes depending on their race, age, and gender identity. The vulnerabilities of their status will result from dynamic processes influenced by group and societal factors and changes in public policy and legislation. A simple change in any facet of identity, such as citizenship status, does not erase additional positional circumstances, which remain enmeshed in a much bigger web of health disparities and systemic failures that also inform social responses to domestic violence.

How one might use the above heuristic will, of course, vary depending on the individual circumstances of the work. We suggest that rhetors engage in co-creation by assessing the "points to consider" and adding or subtracting relevant or irrelevant elements. Conceivably, the same heuristic could be used to frame out the considerations for decision-making in healthcare situations, designing health communications materials and performing an analysis of a specific rhetorical situation. Of course, this heuristic is not simply a tool to effectively address domestic violence discourses. Its general framework can be

TABLE 3.1 A Culture-centered Heuristic for Rhetorical Intervention

	Rhetorical Questions	Points to Consider
Structure	Does this language or analysis reinforce or interrogate existing systems of power and control?	Immigration status Employment status Citizenship
	Which existing social structures constrain or inform rhetorical action in this situation?	Marital status Willingness to invoke police or medical aid
	How might social structures be leveraged or interrogated in this situation?	Access to resources
	Which laws and statutes might apply? How do the people involved understand these laws?	
	Do these structures contribute to marginalizing certain voices and stories? Which ones?	
Culture	Which language(s) are being used in this situation? Are they appropriate for the audience?	Language use (both within and across languages) Vocabulary (plain versus technical language)
	How do the people in this situation identify culturally? What cultural expectations do they bring to the situation?	National identity Religious affiliation
	Which cultures have come into contact in this situation?	Allegiances and antagonisms on a cultural level
	Which cultural stories inform this situation?	Family expectations
	Does the intersection of cultures pose greater or lesser risks for poor consequences? For whom?	
	What are the margins and center of this cultural situation?	
	How do these cultural considerations reflect or reveal systems of power and control?	
Agency	What resources can be accessed? By whom?	Resources available
	What other considerations and obligations might impinge on personal agency?	Power dynamics Finances
	Which decision(s) are possible?	Personal networks and contacts
	How do structures of power and control impact agency?	Insurance

adapted and used for articulating culture-centered information into multiple healthcare contexts as well as the work of rhetorical study. If we return again to the opening exigence of this chapter, that reporting or not reporting domestic violence can be equally potent signals of a need for mental health interventions, one element of concern is the contradictory nature of this communication. Healthcare professionals seeking to identify and help those subject to domestic violence must understand that a lack of communication may itself be a type of communication, perhaps signaling family power structures that prevent calls for help, power outages or failed cell towers.

A culture-centered approach might also go beyond the likely causes of communication or its absence and limit the possibility for a type of inflammatory discourse that creates heightened responses to some situations while masking the importance of others. Culture-centered approaches encourage and require nuanced ways of thinking and therefore avoid simplistic applications of deontological thought that create automatic and categorical responses to single pieces of information. Such a way of thinking, which bioethicist Hilde Lindemann Nelson (2002) might describe as prescriptive and deriving from external principles rather than lived realities, prevents the type of thoughtful rhetorical articulation that can effectively account for historical and other information that differentiates individual rhetorical acts from global dogma. Culture-centered approaches are a potential remedy from this sort of prescription and an invitation into thought. Narrative approaches can help rhetoric and communication scholars identify and tease out the facets of identity considered within an intersection and culture-centered approach, allowing for more effective rhetorical interventions. These points will, of necessity, shift and change in varying situations.

Recursivity and *Mnesis* as Rhetorical Situation Modalities

Although little rhetorical research aside from Nora Augustine's chapter in this volume, has considered domestic violence, such work as exists could easily be incorporated into a culture-centered health communication framework. Drew Holladay's (2017) prior research on post-traumatic stress disorder (PTSD), for instance, considered online groups that could include sufferers of domestic violence diagnosed with PTSD. Individuals negotiating mental health diagnoses must navigate multiple discourses—medical, social, popular—within systems of political and economic power that do not impact all people equally. This work emphasized the psychological impacts of domestic violence, which, as originally detailed in Judith Herman's clinical description of PTSD (1992), hinge on a tension between and ability and an inability to speak. The relationship of domestic violence to all forms of PTSD provides a starting point for culture-centered approaches in this space that could impact healthcare communication as well as rhetorical scholarship.

A crucial concept in rhetorical studies of health and medicine is a construct of "articulation" as both situated and embodied knowledge, notably described by Nathan Stormer (2004) in his well-known working paper on rhetoric and *taxis,* or the arrangement of elements within a text. Articulation, for Stormer, is a performance that must be understood historically, relative to the situatedness of knowledge, a concept he draws from Donna Haraway's extensive body of work. Stormer's essay compellingly illustrates how and why connections between words and things only seem to be necessarily related and that this apparent necessity masks powerful historical and ideological situations that devalue many types of embodied experience. Intersectional and culture-centered approaches are a missing element in the articulation of rhetoric and health communication, especially as they address problems like domestic violence, which occur in family systems embedded in larger cultural matrices, each of which is informed by power structures that disadvantage certain groups. Domestic violence itself, much like the other forms of PTSD that Herman and Holladay discussed, must be understood relative to an intersection of physical and mental assault that complicates each element of intersectional and culture-centered approaches as well as the situatedness of this knowledge. Taking the notion of snapshots Kwame Ture and Charles Hamilton described (1967), each historical moment must be understood in a complex web of relationships that continually changes and evolves.

Stormer's subsequent essay, "Recursivity: A Working Paper on Rhetoric and *Mnesis*" (2013), provides an important assist in describing some barriers to understanding domestic violence in existing rhetorical frameworks. Stormer used domestic violence as a productive example of a situation in which a reminder of past wrong might serve a present purpose in emphasizing the site of absence. When describing an "ability to occupy time" (p. 28) as recursive capacity, Stormer wrote: "discourse about violence constitutes the present ... [which] always becomes the past, hence 'now' is located by 'doing' remembering and forgetting" (p. 28). Ideally, in fact, "recursive modalities may become points of inclusion... enveloping the past through particular balances of memories and amnesias" (p. 45). This notion might seem promising as a modality for rhetorical interventions into domestic violence, as when healthcare workers and carceral authorities rehearse patterns of memory and forgetting that reveal a potential crisis of domestic violence even as it remains hidden and thus outside the reach of public health interventions (Stone, 2020). Yet Stormer seemed to see this ideal as more possible for collective traumatic events enacted in male-dominated and heteronormative settings, noting "the ability to use domestic violence to envelope history in a feminist anti-violence narrative is limited" (p. 45). This potentially disappointing conclusion may be recuperable, however, by recourse to more intersectional and culture-centered approaches.

One problem that might be overcome is Stormer's construction of domestic violence, which parallels that used by the United Nations—as gendered violence between intimate partners, assuming a heteronormative coupling. Stormer cited political action, lawmaking, and television dramas, such as *The Burning Bed,* which illustrate domestic violence as a specific problem of white, heteronormative couplings, making such violence in effect a subversion of the

1950s cult of domesticity. Stormer placed this model of domestic violence in feminist terms, which, as Catherine MacKinnon noted (2013), still require more recourse to intersectional approaches. In effect, Stormer's essay, by using a limited definition of domestic violence, replicated some of the problems noted by Taub (2020) and the APA as affecting successful intervention in domestic violence cases during the COVID-19 stay-at-home orders. If we understand "domestic violence" narrowly and as only impacting certain types of people, then we exclude the majority of those who need help and better access to healthcare.

An objective of the current volume is to identify sites and methods for rhetorical intervention that may effect change in the treatment of mental health both medically and discursively. Since the historical and ideological situations that Stormer (2004) sought to interrogate are themselves culturally informed, they are therefore susceptible to multiple pressures. For instance, the ideology of a "universal woman" that as Lettie Lockhart and Fran Danis (2010) observed, "merely promoted a gender identity and an anti-categorical identity for other socio-political groups" (p. 16), is compatible with Stormer's construction of domestic violence. And as Lockhart and Danis's text emphasized, this universal woman elides existing and experiential facets of personal identity for most women as well as other possible victims of domestic violence. The rhetoric of domestic violence must be situated as cultural and lived identity, yet this project is at odds with the prior history of domestic violence interventions, which reverberate through current experience.

Table 3.2 provides questions intended to help frame a given rhetorical situation against a broader context of how its histories may create sites of recursivity that remain unrecognized. If we consider this type of *mnetic* resituating within health communication—which we define as communications that convey information about individual or community health—as well as communication and rhetorical scholarship, then multiple potential areas for intervention emerge. However, making sense of this information requires further work. For example, highlighting what is remembered and what is forgotten does not provide a necessary site for intervention, but rather illustrates an important context in which an intervention may become possible or necessary. In other words, the situation of remembering and forgetting is not, in itself, an intervention so much as a means of articulating historical information into current circumstances and a means of including such information in current evaluations. Table 3.2, hence, is a useful framework for situating the questions in Table 3.1 within a broader historical framework. However, as these framing questions were designed to encourage culture-centered approaches to recursivity and articulation, the addition of language as a category to consider also provides a platform for adapting our heuristic to additional theoretical models. In other words, the primary framework presented in Table 3.2 can be used to encourage culture-centered approaches to any theoretical position.

TABLE 3.2 Additional Questions for Rhetorical Intervention

	Questions about Historical Articulation	Questions about Recursivity
Structure	What are the origins of these structural circumstances? Is terminology masking structural realities and problems? Which words may be creating confusion or disjunctions in understanding?	Who gets to choose what is remembered and forgotten in this situation? Which societal structures impact access to information about the past?
Culture	What cultural assumptions are held by the most powerful actors in this situation? What are the origins of the cultural stories and assumptions at play? Do past inequities impact this history? Which ones? Can the history of this cultural information provide further helpful information?	What is the past history of interaction between the cultures of the various actors in this situation? Which prior systems of power and control are still exerting an influence in this situation?
Agency	How do personal and cultural histories impact the ability of individuals and communities to recognize their own agency? What limitations exist to claiming agency for the various actors in this situation?	Do prior models of effective agency exist for all of the actors in this situation?
Language	Does the past history of language use the same words to mean the same things? Do historical uses of language exert influence in the current situation?	How might a conflict between past and present communication practices be influencing this situation?

Obstacles to Intervention in the History of Domestic Violence as a Mental Health Issue

As we suggest above, one means of assessing how structure, culture, and agency intersect in current conceptions of domestic violence as a mental health problem is to interrogate the historical origins of the present situation. Such practice is one means of interrogating the power structures and culture that currently limit personal agency. When current experts (Stone, 2020; Taub, 2020) rely on a *mnetic* ability that helps them observe the types of rhetorical absence that Stormer (2013) discussed in terms of domestic violence, they articulate the past into the present. Hence, when Stormer's essay on recursivity situates domestic violence as a site of enveloping history and memory as a means of constructing the present, this recursive capacity includes a past that as Lockhart and Danis (2010) show was already informed by the unhelpful figure of the universal woman. This problematic presence may not be the only invisible historical figure contributing to current inequities. Another problem is a persistently slippery terminology evident in the tendency to consider all domestic violence as heteronormative violence between intimate partners: this problem, too, has a longer history (DeTora, 2010). The single question of past language practice, in fact, can illuminate many potential areas where culture-centered approaches are needed or impeded by unhelpful historical baggage. In examining past language use, additional elements named in Table 3.2 naturally emerge, revealing the origins of culture, structures, and the limits of personal agency.

The origins of language problems regarding domestic violence, in fact, illuminate many different sites of cultural and structural inequities in the current situation. The history of domestic violence as an explicit site of medical and mental health intervention dates to 1962, when such violence was first named, as "battering" (Kempe et al., 1962), a rhetorical move that provides an articulation site for the universal woman as well as the idealized family of the then-popular television situation comedy. The medical discovery of domestic violence as "battering" was a rhetorical maneuver, renaming injuries that until then had been treated in isolation from their causes and termed "undefined trauma" (DeTora, 2010; Gelles & Maynard, 1987; Kempe et al., 1962). As Lisa DeTora previously noted (2010), differences the term "battered" as a diagnostic term applied to young children versus adult women marked a divide in medical versus psychological (and other social science) usages and created rhetorical obstacles to effective healthcare interventions which limited individual agency (Kempe et al., 1962; Walker, 1984); these obstacles have extended into the twenty-first century, creating a need for the intersectional approaches Creshaw (2012) called for. More seriously, the initial publication on battering as a medical and mental health problem created a social structure that conflated clinical practice and juridical intervention, the exact site at which Crenshaw (1991, 2012) called for intersectional approaches.

In "The Battered Child Syndrome," Kempe et al. (1962), pediatric experts in radiology, outlined the rhetorical process by which parents could be convinced to disclose their violent behavior, establishing a medical structure for such encounters. The then-existing structural relationships of parents, children, physicians, and the law shifted profoundly when physicians were enjoined to consult the police, displacing the treatment of injured children into systems of carceral power and thereby reframing battering from a medical problem into a juridical one. The original medical model for treating domestic violence as a medical problem created a power structure that inherently included obstacles to ending, or even discussing, this problem, paralleling the observations in 2020 news coverage and creating the enduring circumstances that Crenshaw (1991,

2012) later cited as endangering families of color disproportionately to other families. And these problems are only compounded for those outside the heteronormative family construction Kempe and colleagues presume.

Hence, the term "battered" took on a gendered meaning in clinical—and specifically mental health—contexts only after it became associated with both police intervention and physical injury. Unlike the battered child, the so-called battered woman was considered to be mentally pathological in seeking domestic violence (DeTora, 2010; Gelles & Maynard, 1987; Herman, 1992; Loseke, Gelles, & Cavanaugh, 2005; Sumter, 2006; Walker, 1984). When psychologist Lenore Walker (1984) interviewed hundreds of women who reported abuse from a husband or boyfriend, however, she learned that these women shared certain psychological symptoms (later grouped with PTSD) only after they had experienced domestic violence (Herman, 1992; Walker, 1984). The clinical structures designed to address the mental health and other impacts of domestic violence on these women also remained independent of the culture-centered questions Dutta (2018) noted as essential to effective healthcare communication (Crenshaw, 1991; DeTora, 2010; Feinberg, 2004; Herman, 1992; Lockhart & Danis, 2010).

Interestingly, the connection of battering, mental pathology, and criminality also underlies the initial clinical descriptions of men who batter their (female) intimate domestic partners. Psychologist Donald Dutton and Susan Golant's (1995) *The Batterer*, the first definitive book-length work describing the psychology of batterers (who are all gender-coded as male), appeared in 1995 and links sociopathy with family violence. Dutton and Golant's work grew out of court-mandated therapy, a circumstance that limited the agency of their patients. The court-mandated treatment also selected for men who had committed egregious acts of violence. In fact, many of the men interviewed were considered guilty of domestic violence because of a general pattern of aggressive and assaultive behavior in other settings. Hence, the initial identification of battering as a clinical problem requiring legal intervention may have reinforced negative physical and mental health impacts, skewing subsequent research and creating obstacles to effective healthcare communication. If we take Crenshaw's (1991) observations about carceral power structures and race into account, then the court-mandated setting of Dutton and Golant's work must be understood, as Dutta suggested, in terms of its uneven application to persons with varying access to power, resources, and agency as well as its focus on men who physically assaulted multiple people and not just family members. Thus, Dutton and Golant's ultimate linkage of psychopathology and sociopathy with battering behavior may have resulted from the characteristics of existing power structures—especially the idea of proof beyond reasonable doubt, which might require additional acts of assault outside the family to corroborate violent personality—rather than clinical reality.

Another linguistic obstacle to culture-centered approaches to domestic violence is the oft-noted circumstance of twentieth-century research: that various phenomena—child abuse, wife abuse, dating violence, husband abuse, elder abuse, same-sex intimate partner abuse, teen abuse, affluent women abuse— were individually discovered and named, reinforcing such violence as simultaneously ubiquitous and unspoken (Abramson, 2020; DeTora, 2010; Dutton & Golant, 1995; Feinberg, 2004; Gelles & Maynard, 1987; Herman, 1992; Kempe et al., 1962; Loseke, Gelles, & Cavanaugh, 2005; Sumter, 2006; Walker, 1984). These discoveries also omitted important sites of domestic conflict and introduced differing terminologies, which left the term "battering" behind in favor of "abuse," creating obstacles to linking these phenomena discursively or seeing family structures rather than individual patients as logical sites for intervention (See Gelles & Maynard, 1987). Although social science and medical research did not explicitly call for rhetorical intervention as such, the shift from terms like "battered woman" to "intimate partner violence" or "family violence," now evident in some settings like the APA website (Abramson, 2020), were intended to break the cycle of endless discovery and to aid in intervention and communication. Yet, as groundbreaking researchers Richard Gelles and Peter Maynard (1987) noted, even after decades of research, categorical thinking about domestic violence limited the ability for meaningful change, even in individual families (Gelles & Cavanaugh, 2005). Lockhart and Danis (2010) continued to work against this unhelpful history to reintegrate all of the facets of identity that characterize the history of intervention into domestic violence.

While culture-centered approaches can help dislodge unspoken ideological constructs like the universal woman from healthcare models and allow communication that accounts for the lived experiences of authentic persons, these experiences must be accessible and legible within the discourse. Intersectionality, similarly, requires attention to multiple facets of being and identity, which can be erased in reductive normative models. As the brief and incomplete history of the term "battering" above shows, models of domestic violence that hinged on heteronormative coupling worked against intersectional modes of understanding domestic violence well after Crenshaw (1991) suggested them in the early 1990s. Multiple discoveries of domestic violence created ironic barriers not only to helping many people but also to understanding domestic violence as embedded within larger social structures. These discoveries came after an initial medical entry that necessarily linked a manifestation of mental illness with the need for carceral interventions. Little wonder that it took some time for domestic violence research to begin to overcome the structural and cultural barriers to taking an intersectional approach to domestic violence, as Lockhart and Danis (2010) showed. Keeping in mind questions like those in Table 3.2 is helpful as a starting point.

Narrative Models for Culture-Centered Interventions

While our heuristics provide a basic framework for information-seeking and decision-making in a given situation, the answers to these questions, considered in isolation, may add to confusion rather than enhancing decision-making or supporting the macro-level changes necessary in our society. Bioethicist Hilde Lindemann Nelson (2002) provided a format for making sense of complex personal circumstances that impact decision-making in clinical healthcare contexts. Nelson's work is predicated on the distinction between narrative approaches to bioethical decision-making in the clinic and an almost juridically conceived model in which the ethicist "acts as a judge, applying lawlike principles derived from one or several of the standing moral theories and using them to prescribe the right course of conduct" (p. 39). In contrast, Nelson provided a more open-ended series of considerations that reside at intersections that are informed by gender, race, and culture and therefore operate by allowing information to flow out of patient and caregiver rather than expecting that standing theories will prescribe conduct. Nelson's model is helpful for addressing the intersectional elements of lived experience and may also be a useful way to convey or organize the information gleaned using the heuristics in Tables 3.1 and 3.2.

Nelson's essay models an ethical decision regarding medical privacy for a patient versus the physical safety and health of a possible caregiver, based on a case gleaned from the bioethics literature. For each subject position within this case, Nelson composes a narrative from that perspective to bring information and inference more clearly into a multifaceted lived context. Nelson's decision framework considers gender, religious belief, access to education, and sexual orientation as important facets of identity that can inform the healthcare decision, a model we see as similar to the heuristic in Table 3.1. Once information is gathered, narratives can be developed from multiple points of view: patient, caregiver, social worker, physician—constructing a series of considerations from varying perspectives. Nelson grounded her discussion in morals and ethics, producing a personalized snapshot of larger systems of power and control within each narrative. In rhetorical research, which often exists outside a specific clinical context directed by a particular medical or treatment decision, further thinking will be needed to identify the best ways to leverage the available information and address pertinent audiences in different research settings and projects.

Multiple areas within rhetorical research can benefit from the approaches we have suggested, especially if we consider these methods as constituting a thinking exercise. The idea of context and sensitive, sustained attention to an intersectional problem may provide even broader applications in the context of the current surge of attention to violence enacted on citizens, particularly persons of color, by carceral authorities. A thoughtful, narrative approach to the rhetorical contexts of domestic violence that mimics Nelson's practice might allow for the articulation of the culture-centered information that would be necessary to meaningfully engage with intersectional identities and situations. And such an approach is important even if the individual narratives and questions only inform (rather than formulate) an end product. Nelson's model of narrative-building also might provide a means of expanding rhetorical interventions beyond immediate situations and into the types of information that would result from the inquiries in Table 3.2. In other words, we see the need for researchers to develop and consider multiple narratives that make sense of domestic violence as an intersectional problem and also take a culture-centered approach to examining this problem and other complex health problems as a long-standing series of historically situated performances played out in varying social and political structures. These narratives, at the least, should be used as a way of thinking through complex problems.

Conclusion

We opened this chapter with the idea that increased attention to domestic violence is needed in RHM work generally and in MHRR specifically. We reviewed several problematic circumstances around the discourse of domestic violence, including its conflation of mental and physical pathology in battered women, conflicting uses of the same term in different settings, and a reliance on specific and unhelpful heterosexually defined gender and family norms. We also examined several approaches to considering, engaging with, or analyzing the discourses of domestic violence: culture-centered communication, intersectionality, narrative bioethics, rhetorical articulation and recursivity. Ultimately, we suggest that effective rhetorical interventions into domestic violence must be intersectional and culture-centered and ought to account for the problems of recursivity we identified, specifically the persistent shadow of the universal woman as the stereotypical figure of domestic violence. Further, we suggest that a recursive approach to narrative-building that accounts for culture, social structures, and agency offers a promising model for ensuring that our interventions account for lived reality and do not revert to unhelpfully stereotypical thinking. We offer heuristics that can be easily adapted to various healthcare, mental health, and social situations as well as rhetorical research and hope that it fosters increased attention to intersectional and cultural identities in future work.

References

Abramson, Ashley. (2020). *How COVID-19 may increase domestic violence and child abuse.* APA Web Site. https://www.apa.org/topics/covid-19/domestic-violence-child-abuse

Andersen, Margaret L., & Collins, Patricia H. (2004). *Race, class, and gender, an anthology* (6th ed.). Wadsworth.

Appleby, George A., Colon, Edgar, & Hamilton, Julia. (2007). *Diversity, oppression, and social functioning* (2nd ed.). Pearson Education.

Collins, Patricia H. (1998). Intersections of race, class, gender, and nation: Some implications for black family studies. *Journal of Comparative Family Studies, 29*(1), 27–36.

Collins, Patricia H. (2000). *Black feminist through: Knowledge, consciousness, and the politics of empowerment* (2nd Ed.). Routledge.

Crenshaw, Kimberlé W. (1991). Mapping the margins: Intersectionality, identity politics, and violence against women of color. *Stanford Law Review, 43*(6), 1241. http://dx.doi.org/10.2307/1229039

Crenshaw, Kimberlé W. (2012). From private violence to mass incarceration: Thinking intersectionally about women, race, and social control. *UCLA Law Review, 59* (1418), 1418–1472.

DeTora, Lisa. (2010). Recognizing the trauma: Battering and the discourse of domestic violence. In Marcelline Block & Angela Laflen (Eds.), *Prescribing gender in medicine and narrative.* Cambridge Scholars Publishing.

Dutta, Mohan J. (2007). Communicating about culture and health: Theorizing culture-centered and cultural sensitivity approaches. *Communication Theory, 17*(3), 304–328.

Dutta, Mohan J. (2008). *Communicating health: A culture-centered approach.* Polity.

Dutta, Mohan J. (2018). Culture-centered approach in addressing health disparities: Communication infrastructures for subaltern voices. *Communication Methods and Measures, 12*(4), 239–259.

Dutton, Donald. G., & Golant, Susan. K. (1995). *The batterer: A psychological profile.* Basic Books.

Feinberg, Cara. (2004). Improvement in the legal response to domestic violence. In Lane E. Volpe (Ed.), *Contemporary issues companion: Battered Women* (pp. 43–74). Greenhaven.

Gelles, Richard, & Maynard, Peter. (1987). A structural family systems approach to intervention in cases of family violence. *Family Relations, 36*(3), 270–275. doi:10.2307/583539

Herman, Judith. (1992). *Trauma and recovery: The aftermath of violence—from domestic abuse to political terror.* Basic Books.

Holladay, Drew. (2017). Classified conversations: Psychiatry and tactical technical communication in online spaces. *Technical Communication Quarterly, 26*(1), 8–24. doi :10.1080/10572252.2016.1257744.

Kempe, C. Henry, Silverman, Frederic N., Steele, Brandt F., Droegemueller, William, & Silver, Henry K. (1962). The battered-child syndrome. *Journal of the American Medical Association, 181*(1), 17–24. doi:10.1001/jama.1962.03050270019004

Lockhart, Lettie L., & Danis, Fran S. (2010). *Domestic violence: Intersectionality and culturally competent practice.* Columbia University Press.

Loseke, Donileen R., Gelles, Richard J., & Cavanaugh, Mary M. (2005). *Current controversies on family violence.* SAGE.

MacKinnon, Catherine. (2013). Intersectionality as method: A note. *Signs, 38*(4), 1019–1030. doi:10.1086/669570

Nelson, Hilde L. (2002). Context: Backwards, sideways, and forward. In Rita Charon & Martha Montello (Eds.), *Stories matter: The role of narrative in medical ethics* (pp. 39–47). Routledge.

Reynolds, J. Fred. (2018). A short history of mental health rhetoric research (MHRR). *Rhetoric of Health & Medicine, 1*(1–2), 1–18.

Sokoloff, Natalie J. (2008). The intersectional paradigm and alternative visions to stopping domestic violence: What poor women, women of color, and immigrant women are teaching us about violence in the family. *International Journal of Sociology of the Family, 34*(2), 153–185.

Spieldenner, Andrew, Robinson, Tomeka M., & Woodruffe, Anjuliet. (2019). The end of AIDS? A critical examination of the National HIV/AIDS Strategy. In Heather

Harris (Ed.), *New-race in the Obama Era* (pp. 93–109). State University of New York Press.

Stone, Alex, Mallin, Alexander, & Gutman, Matt. (2020). Fewer domestic violence calls during COVID-19 outbreak has California officials concerned. *ABC News*. https://abc-news.go.com/US/fewer-domestic-violence-calls-covid-19-outbreak-california/story?id=70336388

Stormer, Nathan. (2004). Articulation: A working paper on rhetoric and *taxis*. *Quarterly Journal of Speech, 90*(3), 257–284.

Stormer, Nathan. (2013). Recursivity: A working paper on rhetoric and *mnesis*. *Quarterly Journal of Speech, 99*(1), 27–50.

Sumter, Melvina. (2006). Domestic violence and diversity: A call for multicultural services. *Journal of Health and Human Services Administration, 29*(2), 173–190.

Taub, Amanda. (2020). A new Covid-19 crisis: Domestic abuse rises worldwide. *New York Times.* https://www.nytimes.com/2020/04/06/world/coronavirus-domestic-violence.html

Ture, Kwame, & Hamilton, Charles V. (1967). *Black power: The politics of liberation.* Random House.

Walker, Lenore. (1984). *The battered woman syndrome.* Springer.

PART II

Legal, Cultural, and Institutional Interventions

4

FACILITATING RHETORIC

Paratherapeutic Activity in Community Support Groups

Nora Augustine

Introduction

In her 2009 memoir *Crazy Love*, an account of her four-year relationship with a physically and emotionally abusive man, Leslie Morgan Steiner described how she gradually rebuilt her life postabuse. Having secured a restraining order and initiated divorce proceedings, Steiner started attending individual psychotherapy twice a week. Her apprehension about this process was manifest: "At the end of every session I expected [my therapist] to proclaim, sadly, that years of therapy were needed to fix me up so I never married a psychopath again" (Steiner, 2010, pp. 290–291). In Steiner's view, her longtime attachment to someone who caused her great harm seemed to be proof of some personal defect on her part; her goal in seeking counseling was, at least implicitly, to transform her whole character from bad to good. Her suggestion that she was broken (needed to be "fixed"), specifically, further conveyed her fears that her abuser had so thoroughly destroyed her emotional health that she would need to rely on therapists to shield her from herself thereafter. Steiner judged herself an object of pity in her therapist's eyes, but she was mistaken—to her surprise, her therapist was optimistic about her future, urging her to speak and write extensively about the life she wanted to live. Ironically, it seems the end result of Steiner's therapy was her recognition that she did not need it as much as she once believed. Although love itself may be "crazy" (as her title suggests), she decidedly was not.

Steiner's self-pathologization may sound harsh to readers, but it is no surprise she once felt this way. According to an unnamed scholar of "batterer" psychology quoted earlier in *Crazy Love*, abusers frequently seek to undermine victims' trust in their own judgments: "He works on her emotionally ... to

DOI: 10.4324/9781003144854-7

make sure she does not tell people about the violence. It's critical that he convinces her the violence is somehow her fault or under her control" (Steiner, 2010, p. 241). The use of crazy-making tactics like gaslighting—in which one party denies another's perceptions of reality (e.g., blaming them for their own abuse)—is a hallmark of interpersonal violence. Such tactics are used to control a person's thoughts and behaviors, including their speech. Thus, it is a commonplace in feminist activism that survivors of gender-based violence benefit from speaking out about their experiences (Alcoff & Gray, 1993).[1] And when survivors speak, it is crucial that their words are believed, respected, and acted on. That is, audiences must grant survivors rhetorical agency, recognizing them as intelligent and rational beings. Yet few would deny trauma carries adverse psychological effects—the most obvious of which is post-traumatic stress disorder (PTSD). For instance, one recent study found that a majority of female survivors of intimate partner violence (IPV) met diagnostic criteria for PTSD; over half were also diagnosable with depression, and nearly one-fifth met criteria for substance abuse disorders (Nathanson et al., 2012). Further muddling the connection between IPV and mental illness, of course, is the fact that some survivors have preexisting psychiatric disorders that are exacerbated, but not created, by their experiences of IPV.

Licensed clinicians and formal psychotherapy play a critical role in helping IPV survivors like Steiner ascertain their need (or not) for long-term psychiatric treatment. Unfortunately, numerous societal, financial, and institutional barriers prevent IPV survivors from utilizing professional mental health services (Rodríguez et al., 2009). Moreover, a rhetorical paradox lies at the center of cultural discourse about IPV, convoluting discussions of real survivors' mental health: should services for those who have experienced trauma construct such persons as psychologically well—or not? In theory, a survivor would benefit from services that engage them as someone who *may* be experiencing a mental health crisis without pathologizing them as someone who *must* be in crisis or (much worse) whose personal psychology is somehow to blame for their predicament. But in practice, where can such ambiguously supportive communications succeed? Who is qualified to support survivors' psychological well-being, and what should they say and do in the process?

Few cultural institutions can speak as well to these questions as the "support group," a concept Rebecca J. Welch Cline (1999) defined as a small number of people who share a "common dilemma" and gather with the goal of providing "mutual aid" (p. 516). Support group participants do not necessarily identify as mental health consumers, and group facilitators are rarely required to be mental health professionals. Yet support groups are inextricably entangled in mental health discourses: the support they offer is implicitly psychological, and their features are consistently described in contrast to—or else collapsed with—those of group psychotherapy. Support groups are also overtly rhetorical. The group's success is judged by how effectively it recognizes each member's "rhetoricity"

(Lewiecki-Wilson, 2003, p. 161), empowering those who have been silenced by trauma to exchange information, empathy, and esteem. The role of a group "facilitator," it follows, is to enable those individual and group communications.

This chapter combines textual analyses of support group literature—specifically, a facilitator training manual—with autoethnographic inquiry to examine the rhetoric of support groups from the perspective of a facilitator. I draw from my subjective experiences as a scholar of mental health rhetoric research (MHRR) and gender studies who has facilitated nearly 170 hours of support groups for fellow IPV survivors at an agency in the southeastern United States. My study attends to popular criticisms of "support" as a misguided intervention that hinders narrative agency, discourages political activism, or otherwise exacerbates the distress it seeks to relieve. Investigating how one agency constructs a facilitator's duties—and reflecting on the experiential knowledge that informs my own practices in that role—I argue that the *paratherapeutic rhetoric* of support groups can serve an essential function in clarifying participants' relationships to mental health. By paratherapeutic rhetoric, I mean communication that looks like therapy, sounds like therapy, has therapeutic aims and/or effects, yet is categorically not therapy. Serving as professional nonprofessionals, support group facilitators possess a liminal status that is especially useful while providing services to trauma survivors. Through rhetorical practices I have labeled as creating space, offering words, and paying forward, facilitators foster conditions under which supportive communication can occur—all without imposing a label of mental illness. In doing so, they affirm the rhetoricity of individuals who have been discredited by an abuser while also serving crucial, if not necessarily clinically significant, mental health needs.

Following a brief review of the rhetoric of support, I describe my involvement with the Compass Center for Women and Families—the IPV agency on which my study is centered.[2] Next, I explicate the three key features introduced above, drawing from my facilitation work and Compass's facilitator training manual to propose the concept of paratherapeutic rhetoric. Ultimately, I suggest that nontraditional care settings like support groups present an unexpected opportunity for MHRR scholar-citizens to partner with social services organizations in our communities. By facilitating rhetoric, or "assembling a public and supporting [their] performances" (Grabill, 2013, p. 193), trained therapeutic practitioners can also facilitate invaluable healing from previously unspoken (or unspeakable) emotional distress.

Who Supports Whom? Overview of Support Groups

What is a support group? Tautologically, it is a group of people who meet to give and/or receive support. As all humans experience adversity, any person could join a support group, and an oft-cited 1994 survey suggested 40% of American adults had participated in one at some time (Wuthnow, 1994).

Scholarship on support groups very often addresses persons coping with cancer, and analyses of online communities are arguably overrepresented in the literature—such public forums are more widely accessible than private, in-person meetings. Indeed, support groups' historic emphasis on anonymity and closed membership may be the greatest obstacle deterring scholars who would study their activities (Helgeson & Gottlieb, 2000, p. 222). Although a group's macrolevel ideology might be available to outsiders, Cline (1999) stressed that "microlevel communication processes"—"actual dialogue, specific messages, and their effects" (p. 521), which are generally unknown to non-attendees—form the substance of a group.

The ambiguity of "support" exacerbates the challenge of explaining what support groups do. Most scholars favor the five dimensions theorized by Carolyn E. Cutrona and Daniel Russell (1990): informational support, emotional support, social integration support, esteem support, and tangible aid (p. 322). Only the last of these locates support in the physical world, and the lack of an action-oriented approach to support forms the basis of many researchers' criticisms of this concept.[3] Support groups, then, are as often defined by what they are *not*—what they do not do—as by what they are.[4] In particular, it is generally agreed that support groups are not therapy: group therapies employ professional psychological assessment, adhere to a fixed schedule, and seek to modify participants' functioning. Put differently, therapy requires an unequal relationship between a facilitator (the locus of accountability) and their clients.[5] On the surface, a support group's operations could be virtually identical to those of group therapy—but it is the facilitator's credentials that officially endow a group with therapeutic value.

Vicki S. Helgeson and Benjamin H. Gottlieb (2000) pointed to the facilitator as the remedy to most of a support group's potential challenges: facilitators are called upon to focus the unfocused, inform the misinformed, hearten the disheartened, and so on (p. 224). Given the diversity of support groups and the spontaneous, collaborative nature of their activities, it is the facilitator—the flesh-and-bone human being, not the abstract concept—who ultimately determines what goes on in any given meeting. It is curious, then, that little scholarship has examined support group communication from a facilitator's perspective. Early ethnographic research on IPV agencies criticized facilitators for distorting clients' accounts and perpetuating stereotypes about abuse (see Loseke, 1992, 2001, 2009), and those findings have often been taken up by later scholars (see Guthrie & Kunkel, 2015; Spencer, 2001). In what follows, I offer an intervention into existing scholarly analyses of support, outlining the methods through which I eventually describe three features of support group communication. Although my own facilitation work grew out of personal and not professional interest, the concept of paratherapeutic rhetoric allows me to articulate both how and why other MHRR scholars might seek to inhabit paratherapeutic roles.

Case Study: The Compass Center for Women and Families

The Compass Center, an agency created through a merger of two nonprofits founded in 1979 and 2000, has served survivors of IPV in Orange County, North Carolina, since 2012.[6] Services range from early prevention of IPV to acute crisis response to long-term, ongoing resources for survivors. Currently, the support group program includes two introductory groups (Domestic Violence I and II) and seven specialized groups: African American-Affirming; DV and Substance Abuse; DV Writing; Latinx-Affirming; LGTBQ-Affirming; Relationship Endings and Healthy Beginnings; and Self-Esteem. Most of Compass's groups meet once a week for 90 minutes (eight weeks total); membership is closed, and members are urged to attend all sessions. An open art-based group called Art of Healing also meets monthly for two hours, and other programming is scheduled as needed. For example, an ad hoc group titled Coping and Stress Management met twice a week from April to June of 2020, addressing the unique stressors of the COVID-19 pandemic. As is common with support groups, prospective members are screened by Compass staff to gauge their current needs, expectations, and possible conflicts of interest.

From November 2014 to April 2016, I participated as a client in four of Compass's support groups: Domestic Violence I, Survivor-Led Writing Group (now DV Writing), a one-off Photovoice project led by graduate students at a nearby university, and several Art of Healing sessions. In May 2016, I answered a call for aspiring facilitators on Compass's support group listserv. The facilitator training program, which I completed in summer 2016, consisted of weekly three-hour sessions (seven weeks total) in which trainees listened to presentations from Compass staff, held small group discussions, and practiced facilitation skills through role-playing exercises—all while following a 90-page training manual.[7] From 2016 until 2018, I intermittently facilitated Art of Healing, eventually leading my first eight-week group (DV Writing) in summer 2018. I facilitated DV Writing again in summer 2019, following this with Self-Esteem in fall 2019; a Holiday Support workshop in December 2019; four Coping and Stress Management sessions in spring 2020; Self-Esteem in summer 2020; Relationship Endings and Healthy Beginnings in fall 2020; a Holiday Support workshop in December 2020; and the LGBTQ-Affirming group in spring 2021.[8] During this time, I also continued to design and lead monthly Art of Healing sessions, and I have facilitated a total of 15 groups for that series.

As of April 2021, I have volunteered about 170 hours with Compass, although this number does not include time spent researching and writing group curricula. My hours of training, practical experience, and independent research in group facilitation have led me to theorize a paratherapeutic rhetoric that strategically "facilitates" supportive communication around experiences of trauma without requiring traumatized persons to identify as mental health consumers. As nontraditional care settings that serve ambiguous mental health needs, support groups expand popular understandings of who wields power over whose rhetoricity (and how) in times of severe psychological distress, demanding further inquiry from MHRR scholars.

Paratherapeutic Rhetoric in Theory and Practice

In this section, I draw on my facilitation work and the Compass Center's 2019 facilitator manual to sketch three features of support group rhetoric, suggesting the term "paratherapeutic rhetoric" for the communication that occurs in Compass's groups.[9] The prefix "para-" is suitably expansive, meaning "analogous or parallel to, but separate from or going beyond," the word it modifies (Para-, 2005). When I refer to paratherapeutic rhetoric, I mean communications that are "analogous or parallel to" professional therapeutic practices while also being distinctly "separate from or going beyond" the same.[10] As I noted above, support consists in communicative acts, and the success of a support group hinges on its participants' rhetorical abilities. Through paratherapeutic rhetorical practices, I argue, facilitators strategically blur boundaries between clients' communication in support groups and that which they would have with therapists, educators, or friends and family. It is through this blurring that other crucial information might become clearer: support groups recover the rhetorical authority that clients' abusers have (in a sense) stolen from them, offering relief while valuably clarifying their interest in more formal psychiatric labels and treatments. Using data from a textual analysis of Compass's facilitator manual and deep autoethnographic inquiry, I propose below three strategies through which support group leaders enact both individual and collective rhetoricity. These are, in my chosen nomenclature: creating space, offering words, and paying forward.

Creating Space

Literally and figuratively, an IPV agency should be a space that invites communication. Measures taken to make Compass accessible to clients—all of its services are free, most are available in Spanish, in-house childcare is provided, and so on (Compass, 2019, p. 4, 10)—have obvious practical value, minimizing barriers to clients' participation. They also build Compass's credibility, demonstrating the agency's desire to serve diverse survivors with concrete resources. But perhaps the most powerful way in which Compass creates space for clients' communications is by its very existence: it is a physical location with locked doors that separate occupants from the outside world. This is a building for which, essentially, there is no other purpose but to engage in supportive communication around IPV. At the same time, because support groups are only one of many services Compass recommends to clients, the needs they meet are implicitly likened to the more overt, concrete impacts of abuse that the agency addresses through things like career counseling, legal advice, and housing assistance. Supportive communication is thus positioned as not only a normal part of the healing process but also as tangible aid to which clients are entitled—it is something they *may* need, although it is not something they *must* need.

Walking down the mostly residential street on which Compass is located, one could easily mistake the large Colonial Revival–style house for a local family's home. Upon entering the agency, one encounters a plush couch, armchairs, fluffy throw pillows, a coffee table covered in magazines, and an assortment of homey knickknacks. The carpeted, den-like rooms in which groups convene are similarly adorned. Clients are offered a drink or snack, sometimes fetching these themselves from a room indistinguishable from any other household kitchen but for the industrial multifunction printer in one corner. Boxes of tissues abound in every room, clearly signaling the normalcy of crying here. In sum, whereas prevailing images of "support groups" show something like a circle of folding chairs in a bare, sterile room (e.g., a school gym), Compass's appearance straddles that of a therapist's office and the authentic domestic settings such offices seek to mimic. As a visual form of paratherapeutic rhetoric, the agency's resemblance to both of these places signals its provision of a space that is simultaneously public and private—the discussions that occur therein can be as professional or as personal as visitors choose, and those choices can be modified at any time.

Through the specified work of support groups, facilitators expand upon the visual and written rhetorics of healing that characterize Compass's self-presentation as a whole. On the first day of a group, facilitators circulate brightly colored pocket folders that contain pregroup paperwork, a schedule of activities, and relevant handouts. In the groups I have led, clients also received brand-new notebooks of varying styles, and writing utensils are dispersed throughout the room. Clearly, the presence of these supplies is meant to encourage clients to translate their subjective thoughts and feelings into written words; they also allow group members to express their individuality through the choice of one design over another, and their quality speaks to the dignity with which Compass aims to treat its clients. In keeping with Compass's presentation as a home-away-from-home, clients are invited to store their group materials at the agency if they are wary of items getting lost or intruded upon elsewhere. Finally, each new Compass group starts with clients signing a standardized "Participation Agreement" in which they pledge to attend and participate in the group to the best of their abilities (Compass, 2019, p. 84). Signing this (nonbinding) paperwork is a means of concretizing our collective commitment to the group and openly affirming our desire to give and take support in this setting. Whereas clients may enter Compass as visitors, passively receiving services from the staff, their acts of choosing and using these materials mark them as active cocreators of the support group space.

Beyond the administrative tasks that preface each Compass group, facilitators employ several introductory activities that help create a space conducive to supportive communication. Two that feature prominently in facilitator training are (1) group guidelines and (2) mindfulness exercises. As the first activity performed in the first meeting of a group, the establishment of group guidelines is explicitly intended to urge clients to "share their opinions and arguments" and "allow for open sharing, even with differences of opinion" (Compass, 2019, p. 84, 76). Facilitators suggest a few ground rules for our discussions—for example, confidentiality ("What is said in the group stays in the group") and respect ("We respect others' differences, beliefs, lifestyles … etc.")—and ask the group to build from these (Compass, 2019, p. 83). Clients' responses are handwritten on an oversized sticky note, which is reposted in subsequent sessions for our reference and revision (Compass, 2019, p. 84). Some guidelines are easily agreed upon: clients might forbid interruptions, harsh judgment of others' healing processes, or unsolicited advice (solicited is usually okay). Other topics, such as the type of language we will permit, may be more controversial: whereas some clients strongly desire to use curse words to express authentic emotions, those who have endured verbal abuse may find the same words distressing. Nonetheless, our discussions are more often concerned with specifying things that *are* acceptable during our group sessions than those that are not. Welcoming diverse habits of thought, feeling, and language, the group guidelines encourage us to recognize ourselves and one another as basically well-intentioned people with valuable things to say. Moreover, in the process of constructing our collective answer to the question, "How do I want to be spoken to?" group participants are also individually challenged to consider, "How do I want to speak?"

The use of mindfulness activities at Compass further fosters the conditions in which clients might actively participate in support group discussions. Quoting influential work by Jon Kabat-Zinn (1994), Compass's facilitator manual characterized mindfulness as "paying attention in a particular way: on purpose, in the present moment, and nonjudgmentally" (2019, p. 43). A notable benefit of mindfulness is that it "Helps you become more fully engaged in activities … [and] really participate in one thing fully" (Compass, 2019, p. 43).[11] By opening every group session with a directed mindfulness exercise, facilitators seek to unite a cluster of near-strangers from all walks of life into a cohesive group with shared experiences, values, and goals. The exercises—which facilitators may read from a script, play from a recording, or spontaneously improvise based on prior knowledge—are meant to be physically and mentally calming, prompting us to set aside our daytime stressors and symbolically cross over into the group's space and time. Importantly, facilitators are not called upon to name the source of clients' stress or the central topic to which we should direct our focus, for each group member has already disclosed their status as an IPV survivor (and a person seeking support) by virtue of showing up. To promote communication, facilitators work to welcome clients into a space where it is possible both to speak about one's traumas and, once having spoken, not to be defined by those traumas. The paratherapeutic function of creating space, then, is not that these practices urge us to discuss abuse per se, but rather that they urge us to discuss what we actually want to discuss.

Offering Words

The Compass Center's group curricula draw from diverse sources—scholars, activists, clinicians, artists, and more—and our exploration of these materials in each group meeting surely constitutes what Cutrona and Russell (1990) called "informational support" (p. 322), or practical guidance for understanding a dilemma. That facilitators share facts and model healing behaviors is a given for many scholars of support (Helgeson & Gottlieb, 2000, p. 239), but it should be clarified that facilitators also offer a vocabulary and rhetorical frameworks for clients' use in articulating their experiences. Make no mistake: the facilitator's job is not to tell clients what to think or say, but rather to "facilitate" the circumstances under which they can say what they already think (or know intuitively). In this sense, IPV support groups might be likened to feminist consciousness-raising groups of the 1960s and onwards—they are semi-public forums for situating deceptively private issues within their broader cultural, political, and discursive contexts. Specifically, Compass's facilitator manual described its groups as "psychoeducational" (2019, p. 6), elsewhere citing a source that defined the "primary focus" of psychoeducational groups as: "to provide education and support, and to increase knowledge and coping skills. ... [It] is hoped that those who attend psychoeducational support groups learn information to increase their functioning in the world" (Washington Coalition of Sexual Assault Programs, 2014, p. 11). By their very nature, Compass's groups are meant to educate clients about psychological matters, engaging them in communicative acts that are as intellectually precise as they are emotionally supportive. Perhaps this is why, in my experience, it is not uncommon for clients to refer to our weekly support group meetings as "classes" or to the group itself as a "class."

As Compass is an IPV agency, one word we inevitably offer for debate in its support groups is "abuse," especially as this label is applied to nonphysical violence. Who can say they were abused, and what is the rhetorical import of doing so? The Power and Control Wheel is a landmark tool created by Domestic Abuse Intervention Programs for the express purpose of filling a void in cultural discourse about "battering" (2017, para. 1). It lists over 50 words and phrases one might use to describe an abuser's actions. Compass's adapted version of the Wheel, printed in the facilitator manual, divided the Wheel's items into eight key categories: "Using intimidation," "Emotional abuse," "Using isolation," "Denying, minimizing, blaming," "Using children," "Using privilege," "Economic abuse," and "Using coercion & threats" (Compass, 2019, p. 34). To my knowledge, every support group at Compass reviews the Power and Control Wheel at some point; facilitators frequently ask group members to read the Wheel aloud and compare its terminology against their own experiences. Of course, the point of doing this is not to inform clients that they may have been abused—they would not be at Compass if they did not already know this. In this paratherapeutic setting, the Wheel rather offers names for abuse that has already occurred, highlighting the strategic (i.e., power-seeking) aspects of abusers' behaviors. For instance, "Displaying weapons" and "Smashing things" are deciphered as forms of intimidation, "Interfering with work or education" as economic abuse, "gaslighting/playing mind games" as emotional abuse, and so on (Compass, 2019, p. 34). By drawing from the Power and Control Wheel and its counterpart, the Equality Wheel (for healthy relationships), facilitators explicitly invite clients to name and frame their experiences as either the presence of abuse or the absence of equality. In the process, group members might be assured that their subjective pain is, in fact, an objectively appropriate response to their experiences—regardless of whether they choose to label and/ or relieve that pain through professional means.

As facilitators offer words to clients, the skill of "active listening," which involves "Using your words to say what you think the person has said" and "asking if you understood correctly," serves three key functions (Compass, 2019, p. 16). First, the back-and-forth structure of this practice naturally urges clients to share more and more about themselves: per Compass's facilitator manual, active listening should be used "when you want the person to keep talking with you" (2019, p. 20). Second, active listening effectively workshops both parties' language choices, closing the gap between the speaker's meaning and the listener's perceptions. By reflecting the content of clients' comments and imagining the emotions that may be driving them—for example, by saying, "From your tone of voice, you seem to be feeling [blank] … does that seem true?" (Compass, 2019, p. 21, ellipsis in original)—facilitators literally offer words for clients to accept, reject, or modify as needed. Third, active listening allows for "ventilation" in a crisis, helping speakers purge raw emotions (since "feelings are transient and can be illogical") and make room for more deliberative "problem solving" (Compass, 2019, p. 23). Indeed, the facilitator manual emphasized that "The most important step in Crisis Intervention is Active Listening. This may be all you do. DO NOT RUSH too quickly into problem solving" (2019, p. 24). Active listening is valued precisely because it is not action-oriented; it rather "encourage[s] clients to utilize inner resources and … arrive at their own best answers" (Compass, 2019, p. 22).

The sections of Compass's facilitator manual that address "Crisis Intervention" and "Suicide Intervention" undoubtedly convey the psychological gravity of a facilitator's work (2019, pp. 22–24, 32). Accordingly, I would be remiss to understate support groups' reliance on formal psychiatric discourse. Discussions of PTSD, depression, substance abuse, and other mental health issues are all but bound to surface in any gathering of trauma survivors. But notably, it is not just Compass's clients' mental health that may be lamented or defended in our meetings: their abusers' psyches are also closely scrutinized. Per the facilitator manual, common abuser characteristics such as "hypersensitivity" and a "Dr. Jekyll/Mr. Hyde personality" ("explosiveness and moodiness") may cause "The survivor [to] think the abuser has some sort of mental problem" (Compass, 2019, p. 37); threats of suicide are also a very common abusive tactic (Compass, 2019, p. 34). The manual did not mention "narcissism," a word that carries increasingly pathological connotations, but I am certain I have heard clients assign this quality to abusers more often than any other. It is a mark of support groups' distinctly paratherapeutic aims that clients might simultaneously describe an abuser as "crazy," "insane," "psycho," and so on—words that noticeably perpetuate ableism against persons with mental illness—while also identifying themselves as potential consumers of psychiatric care. Clearly, trauma survivors find it meaningful to explore how traumatic events are connected to mental health, pondering the psychological processes that might allow someone to inflict or endure severe interpersonal violence. Psychiatric terms may not be words a paratherapeutic practitioner offers, then, but in order to engage in active listening around trauma, they are words we need to know.

In a section of Compass's facilitator manual titled "Common Mental Health Disorders," the agency affirmed that "it is important for facilitators to be aware" of common psychiatric symptoms and treatments "so they can help support clients in group"—and notify Compass staff of any crisis situations (Compass, 2019, p. 26).[12] But as one would expect, Compass also sharply contrasted support groups with therapy at various points, stressing that group facilitators "are not mental health professionals" and "we are not here to treat mental illness" (2019, p. 26; see also p. 12, 95).[13] These recurring statements not only fulfill an obvious ethical imperative; they imply that, without such disclaimers, Compass's support groups would be therapeutically ambiguous (so to speak). And they would—many volunteer facilitators *are* also professional counselors, and many clients are mental health consumers. Exchanges between those parties might represent the purest form of paratherapeutic rhetoric, but we still would not assert that support groups are "therapy," because doing so carries acute potential for harm in this particular setting. Indeed, a defining feature of paratherapeutic rhetoric often seems to be that, the closer our communication verges on actual therapy, the more vital it is that we are emphatically not in therapy. Compass noted that the benefits of an IPV support group include "Counteract[ing] self-blame," "De-pathologizing," and "Confirm[ing] experience" (2019, p. 13). Citing both scientific facts and experiential knowledge, groups collectively argue that their experiences of IPV and its sequelae do not make them masochistic, sick, crazy, or otherwise deviant. If they choose to access formal mental health services, it is not because, as Steiner wrote in *Crazy Love*, "years of therapy are needed to fix [them] up" (2009, p. 290). Thus, the words a facilitator does not offer are just as crucial as the ones they do: we are not there to diagnose or treat clients' (or abusers') mental illnesses. As paratherapeutic practitioners, we are there to support their rhetorical performances, listening while they themselves gradually clarify what "mental health" might mean to them.

Paying Forward

Outside of Compass, confidentiality is probably the most critical duty of the support group facilitator role. But inside Compass, the facilitator manual noted, facilitators "will make the most use of respect, genuineness, and empathy [skills]" (Compass, 2019, p. 50). Notice that, whereas respect and empathy entail some amount of deliberative thought, genuineness implies the absence of the same—it is better described as a way of being, "demonstrated by congruency between the many different elements of your communication" such that "you are likely to be seen as believable" (Compass, 2019, p. 49). Irrespective of what a facilitator actually says in a support group, clients are unlikely to open up about experiences of trauma if they do not believe the facilitator has their best interests at heart. For this reason, facilitators use a range of rhetorical strategies to identify themselves as both givers and, importantly, receivers of genuine kindness. This paying forward, as I call it, is a means of building a distinctly paratherapeutic facilitator-client relationship—one that, although it does not technically confer therapeutic benefits, is no less grounded in serious mutual concern about trauma, mental health, and healing.

In Compass's facilitator manual, the ability to facilitate support groups (specifically, through active listening) was defined as "a communication skill," and "Like all other skills, it takes practice" (2019, p. 20). Compass stressed that supportive communication is not an intrinsic talent, but rather a challenge that facilitators must be motivated to attempt over and over again until they finally excel at it. In short, to be an effective support group facilitator, one must truly want to facilitate support. Among several "Preferred Characteristics and Background[s]" in the facilitator manual's "Volunteer Position Description," four pointed to the facilitator's presumed altruism: "advocacy experience in the [IPV] field" "previous experience … leading support groups or group therapy," "cultural competence with diverse populations," and "a passion for helping and supporting others" (Compass, 2019, p. 6). Noting that facilitators are held to a "high standard," the manual assigned "utmost importance" to facilitators' own investment in their work—volunteers are urged to study their strengths and weaknesses "so they can continue challenging themselves to live up to their full potential" (Compass, 2019, p. 58). Once again, Compass stressed the centrality of "authentic and sincere expression" in perfecting facilitation skills: "the ability to give group members truthful and sincere feedback is very important … [this] includes providing comments from a place of authenticity and a sincere interest in promoting group members' well-being" (2019, p. 58). Through repeated displays of genuineness and a related skill, "Self-Disclosure" (Compass, 2019, p. 49), facilitators slowly earn the group's trust in their good intentions, encouraging clients to respond with their own honest reflections.

Since facilitators serve Compass's clients directly, holding a position of trust with IPV survivors, it is certainly reasonable for the agency to expect them to be decent people. But from a facilitator's perspective, how exactly does one convey one's good intentions to clients? It goes without saying, I suppose, that the foremost way in which Compass's facilitators show their commitment to paratherapeutic practice is by volunteering in the first place: even those who are professional therapists are not paid for their labor in support groups, and clients are generally aware of this. One of the most compelling choices a support group facilitator can make, too, is to disclose their own experiences of trauma. In my experience, a large majority of Compass's facilitators are either survivors of abuse/assault—if not former Compass clients—or they have a close relationship with someone who is.[14] That facilitators who self-identify as trauma survivors might be "paying it forward" with their volunteer work, performing acts of kindness for others that are similar to those which they once received in a time of need, could not be clearer in the support group setting. But the idea that self-disclosure promotes supportive communication is plausible for numerous reasons: it illuminates a facilitator's motives, lends credence to displays of empathy, builds intimacy through mutual vulnerability, and so on. When the line between so-called leaders and followers is suspended, all participants might speak more freely in the group's discussions, since no one is bound to the dichotomous roles of "battered woman" versus "strong and independent woman" that Donileen Loseke (1992) rightly criticized (p. 100).

Importantly, the scene I am describing may be therapeutic, but it is not therapy. Therapists are discouraged from confiding in clients about personal matters. Even if their practice seeks to modify behavior, the goal is not for clients to be more like therapists. And the goal of Compass's groups is not for clients to become volunteers, either—but if the group functions as expected, clients will start "Assuming some facilitator functions," introducing new topics and feedback in group sessions and prompting others to do the same (Compass, 2019, p. 72). After all, a cornerstone of support group ideology is the "helper-therapy principle," or the belief that members benefit as much (or more) from helping others as they do from being helped (Riessman, 1965, p. 27). If supportive communication begets healing, and healing begets a "desire to work for the battered women's movement" (e.g., by promoting others' rhetoricity in future support groups) (Winkelmann, 2004, p. 210), then paratherapeutic rhetoric in the form of paying forward is both a means to an end and an end in itself.

Conclusion: Mental Health Rhetoric and Being Useful

It is likely that the problematic trends scholars once observed in the practice of "support"—and facilitators' actions in particular—are slowly improving as popular and scholarly understandings of trauma progress. Research on the rhetoric of support groups is incipient, and I do not assert that my personal experience at Compass is any more accurate, representative, or fascinating than other qualitative studies of IPV services. Nevertheless, what my findings absolutely share with Loseke's (1992) trailblazing work is the conviction that, even at times when supportive communication has failed to recognize clients' rhetoricity, the facilitator probably meant well: they "understood themselves as helping clients do what they *had to do* and there was a moral rightness to their position," even if the outcome was wholly wrong (p. 113).

Lest I sound dreadfully self-righteous, I stress that I facilitate support groups at Compass in part because I feel deeply indebted to this agency—and I benefit from the helper-therapy principle, too. Hence, it is on this point of personal relevance and public service that I wish to conclude my discussion in this chapter. In his brief history of MHRR, J. Fred Reynolds (2018) observed that scholarship in this subfield has "almost always been prompted, at least initially, by coincidental friend/family/personal connections to the world of mental health" (p. 3). For example, Reynolds mentioned that Kimberly Emmons's (2010) illuminating monograph, *Black Dogs and Blue Words*, was partially inspired by her past volunteer work with "a local NAMI office" (Reynolds, 2018, p. 9). If a goal of MHRR is to intervene in current practices for serving persons in distress, then we might search for them in nontraditional care settings. Participating in support groups is common; all humans are in need of "support" at one time or another, and those needs cannot always be met through formal psychiatric treatment. Through further analysis of the features, functions, and even dangers of paratherapeutic communication in support groups, MHRR stands to make a tangible contribution to our fellow citizens' mental health. As members of a discipline "in the midst of discovering anew its usefulness" in public life (Coogan & Ackerman, 2013, p. 1), rhetoricians might be exactly what community nonprofits are looking for to support their work in ways yet untold—and I hope we let ourselves be found.

Notes

1 The preferred term for someone who has experienced traumatic violence is its own rhetorical conundrum. For the sake of simplicity, I default to the common words "survivor" and (most often) "client" in this chapter, though I am wary of both terms.
2 The analyses in this chapter are necessarily limited, and they are entirely my own: I do not speak on behalf of the Compass Center or its clients in any way.
3 Dana Cloud (1998), for one, argued that compulsory media "support" for U.S. troops and families during the Persian Gulf War displaced legitimate political unrest by framing it as personal, emotional problems (p. 87). Similarly, Val Gillies

(2005) and Gretchen Brion-Meisels (2014) showed how institutional "support" for (respectively) vulnerable students in the American school system or marginalized parents under British family policy failed to consider the complex sociocultural factors informing each group's actual needs. According to these scholars and others, support might be viewed as a theoretical construct that persons with power invoke to placate others in distress while apparently declining to relieve that distress with tangible aid.

4 Helgeson and Gottlieb (2000) contrasted support groups with self-help groups, arguing that the former have more "uniformity and structure" in their membership, number/length of meetings, reliance on professionals, and "advocacy activities" (p. 222). On the other hand, Shelley E. Taylor (2011) called self-help groups "a particular type of social support group" (p. 205), and Cline (1999) asserted that "most scholars use these terms interchangeably" (p. 519).

5 Cline (1999) listed seven qualities that differentiate support groups from group therapy, and nearly all of these are linked to the unequal relationship between therapists and clients: "(a) institutional affiliation, fees, appointments, and records; (b) a clinical environment; (c) a high degree of structure; (d) preset agendas for changing behavior; (e) status differentiation between professionals and clients; (f) unilateral self-disclosure by clients and social support from professionals; (g) therapists as authorities" (p. 519).

6 Compass generally uses the term "domestic violence" in their support group program, conveying that they serve survivors of family violence as well as persons who have experienced abuse from a romantic partner. The word "domestic" is not meant to exclude clients who have never cohabited with their abusers; likewise, "violence" is absolutely not limited to physical violence. I have chosen to use the umbrella term "intimate partner violence" (IPV) in this chapter, because the bulk of my work with Compass has focused on this particular type of abuse.

7 Four of these training sessions were conducted jointly with staff and trainees from a local rape crisis center due to the obvious overlap in the skill sets needed to facilitate groups at these two organizations. Newly-trained facilitators are also encouraged to shadow a current facilitator during a one-day session before they begin to sign up for eight-week groups, and when someone facilitates their first group, they are paired with an experienced volunteer.

8 Although I use the unprefixed verb "facilitate" throughout this chapter, I wish to stress that Compass's groups are always assigned two co-facilitators—we never work alone. Additionally, I should clarify that from March 2020 to my time of writing, all of Compass's support groups have convened via Zoom due to the COVID-19 pandemic.

9 The 2019 edition of the training manual is nearly identical to the one I used in 2016, which I still have in my possession. I cite the most recent version to confirm (and ensure) that my study is up-to-date.

10 The term "paratherapeutic" has been used sparingly by psychologists, often denoting treatments that operate alongside individual psychotherapies. For example, Luciano L'Abate (1991) argued that paratherapeutic writing assignments could supplement the actual therapy clients receive in face-to-face appointments (p. 88). Many thanks are due to my colleague, Tyler Easterbrook, for suggesting the prefix "para-" to me. I much prefer this to several possible alternatives (e.g., "semi-," "quasi-", "pseudo-," etc.).

11 The set of beliefs and practices now commonly referred to as "mindfulness meditation" has grown increasingly popular in Western therapies, self-help books/groups, offices, schools, and various other contexts since Kabat-Zinn first popularized this concept in the United States. Having reached peak popularity around 2014 (Walsh, 2016, p. 153), mindfulness practices have since become a subject of considerable controversy; their therapeutic effects are disputed. For some influential discussions

of mindfulness and its critiques by social scientists, see (e.g.) Barker (2014), Harrington and Dunne (2015), Hickey (2010), Walsh (2016), etc.

12 Compass policy explicitly requires volunteers to notify staff if, for example, a client "tell[s] us that they're going to hurt themselves or someone else, or if a minor [or disabled adult] is in danger" (Compass, 2019, p. 22).

13 Notably, this sentence is one of very few in Compass's manual that is fully underlined for emphasis.

14 Given that nearly all of the Compass Center's facilitators are women—as are the clients, although Compass's services are open to survivors of all identities—it is unsurprising that a significant portion of them have experienced some form of violence in their lives.

References

Alcoff, Linda, & Gray, Laura. (1993). Survivor discourse: Transgression or recuperation? *Signs: Journal of Women in Culture and Society, 18*(2), 260–290. https://doi.org/10.1086/494793

Barker, Kristin K. (2014). Mindfulness meditation: Do-it-yourself medicalization of every moment. *Social Science & Medicine, 106,* 168–176. https://doi.org/10.1016/j.socscimed.2014.01.024

Brion-Meisels, Gretchen. (2014). The challenge of holistic student support: Investigating urban adolescents' constructions of support in the context of school. *Harvard Educational Review, 84*(3), 314–340.

Cline, Rebecca J. Welch. (1999). Communication within social support groups. In Lawrence R. Frey, Dennis S. Gouran, & Marshall Scott Poole (Eds.), *The handbook of group communication theory and research* (pp. 516–538). SAGE Publications.

Cloud, Dana L. (1998). *Control and consolation in American culture and politics: Rhetoric of therapy.* SAGE Publications.

Compass Center for Women and Families. (2019). *Support group facilitator training manual.* Compass Center for Women and Families.

Coogan, David J., & Ackerman, John M. (2013). Introduction: The space to work in public life. In John M. Ackerman & David J. Coogan (Eds.), *The public work of rhetoric: Citizen-scholars and civic engagement* (pp. 1–16). University of South Carolina Press.

Cutrona, Carolyn E., & Russell, Daniel Wayne. (1990). Type of social support and specific stress: Toward a theory of optimal matching. In Barbara R. Sarason, Irwin G. Sarason, & Gregory R. Pierce (Eds.), *Social support: An interactional view* (pp. 319–366). J. Wiley & Sons.

Domestic Abuse Intervention Programs. (2017). *Understanding the Power and Control Wheel.* https://www.theduluthmodel.org/wheels/faqs-about-the-wheels/

Emmons, Kimberly. (2010). *Black dogs and blue words: Depression and gender in the age of self-care.* Rutgers University Press. http://public.eblib.com/choice/publicfullrecord.aspx?p=868537

Gillies, Val. (2005). Meeting parents' needs? Discourses of "support" and "inclusion" in family policy. *Critical Social Policy, 25*(1), 70–90. https://doi.org/10.1177/0261018305048968

Grabill, Jeffrey T. (2013). On Being Useful: Rhetoric and the Work of Engagement. In John M. Ackerman & David J. Coogan (Eds.), *The public work of rhetoric: Citizen-scholars and civic engagement* (pp. 193–208). University of South Carolina Press.

Guthrie, Jennifer A., & Kunkel, Adrianne. (2015). Problematizing the uniform application of the formula story: Advocacy for survivors in a domestic violence support group. *Women and Language, 38*(1), 43–62.

Harrington, Anne, & Dunne, John D. (2015). When mindfulness is therapy: Ethical qualms, historical perspectives. *American Psychologist, 70*(7), 621–631. https://doi.org/10.1037/a0039460

Helgeson, Vicki S., & Gottlieb, Benjamin H. (2000). Support groups. In Sheldon Cohen, Lynn G. Underwood, Benjamin H. Gottlieb, & Fetzer Institute (Eds.), *Social support measurement and intervention: A guide for health and social scientists* (pp. 221–245). Oxford University Press.

Hickey, Wakoh Shannon. (2010). Meditation as medicine: A critique. *CrossCurrents, 60*(2), 168–184. https://doi.org/10.1111/j.1939-3881.2010.00118.x

Kabat-Zinn, Jon. (1994). *Wherever you go, there you are: Mindfulness meditation in everyday life* (1st ed). Hyperion.

L'Abate, Luciano. (1991). The use of writing in psychotherapy. *American Journal of Psychotherapy, 45*(1), 87–98. https://doi.org/10.1176/appi.psychotherapy.1991.45.1.87

Lewiecki-Wilson, Cynthia. (2003). Rethinking rhetoric through mental disabilities. *Rhetoric Review, 22*(2), 156–167.

Loseke, Donileen R. (1992). *The battered woman and shelters: The social construction of wife abuse.* State University of New York Press.

Loseke, Donileen R. (2001). Lived realities and formula stories of "battered women." In Jaber F. Gubrium & James A. Holstein (Eds.), *Institutional selves: Troubled identities in a postmodern world* (pp. 107–126). Oxford University Press.

Loseke, Donileen R. (2009). Public and personal stories of wife abuse. In Evan Stark & Eva Schlesinger Buzawa (Eds.), *Violence against women in families and relationships* (pp. 1–36). Praeger/ABC-CLIO.

Nathanson, Alison M., Shorey, Ryan C., Tirone, Vanessa, & Rhatigan, Deborah L. (2012). The prevalence of mental health disorders in a community sample of female victims of intimate partner violence. *Partner Abuse, 3*(1), 59–75. https://doi.org/10.1891/1946-6560.3.1.59

Reynolds, J. Fred. (2018). A short history of mental health rhetoric research (MHRR). *Rhetoric of Health & Medicine, 1*(1–2), 1–18. https://doi.org/10.5744/rhm.2018.1003

Riessman, Frank. (1965). The "helper" therapy principle. *Social Work, 10*(2), 27–32.

Rodríguez, Michael, Valentine, Jeanette M., Son, John B., & Muhammad, Marjani. (2009). Intimate partner violence and barriers to mental health care for ethnically diverse populations of women. *Trauma, Violence, & Abuse, 10*(4), 358–374. https://doi.org/10.1177/1524838009339756

Spencer, J. William. (2001). Self-presentation and organizational processing in a human service agency. In Jaber. F. Gubrium & James A. Holstein (Eds.), *Institutional selves: Troubled identities in a postmodern world* (pp. 158–175). Oxford University Press.

Steiner, Leslie Morgan (2010). *Crazy love: A memoir.* St. Martin's Press.

Taylor, Shelley E. (2011). Social support: A review. In Howard S. Friedman (Ed.), *The Oxford handbook of health psychology* (pp. 189–214). Oxford University Press.

Walsh, Zack. (2016). A meta-critique of mindfulness critiques: From McMindfulness to critical mindfulness. In Ronald E. Purser, David Forbes, & Adam Burke (Eds.), *Handbook of Mindfulness* (pp. 153–166). Springer International Publishing. https://doi.org/10.1007/978-3-319-44019-4_11

Washington Coalition of Sexual Assault Programs. (2014). *Circle of hope: A guide for conducting psychoeducational support groups* (2nd ed.). Washington Coalition of Sexual Assault Programs. https://www.wcsap.org/sites/default/files/uploads/working_with_survivors/support_groups/Circle_of_Hope_2014.pdf

Winkelmann, Carol L. (2004). *The language of battered women: A rhetorical analysis of personal theologies.* State University of New York Press.

Wuthnow, Robert. (1994). *Sharing the journey: Support groups and the quest for a new community.* Free Press. http://www.myilibrary.com?id=899034

5

WOMEN OF DIGNITY AND GRACE

The Politics of Respectability in Alcoholics Anonymous

Lori J. Joseph and Stephanie Kelley-Romano

Introduction

Alcoholism, or alcohol use disorder (AUD) is a significant public health problem in the United States. It is estimated that 20 million Americans have some form of substance use disorder, and a full 15 million people suffer from AUD. Despite spending billions of dollars on healthcare, and losing millions in lost work, the National Institute on Alcohol Abuse and Alcoholism (NIAAA) estimates that there are approximately 95,000 deaths per year attributed to alcohol misuse (Alcohol Facts and Statistics, 2021). Because of the COVID-19 pandemic and resulting lockdowns, these numbers are on the rise. A recent study by William Killgore found that for those under lockdown, "hazardous alcohol use rose from 21% in April to 40.7% in September" (Murez, 2021). Therefore, "the alcohol problem" seems to show no signs of abating.

There are a variety of approaches to treating AUD, including: group psychotherapy with moderating approaches, mutual-aid support groups which focus on moderating drinking, medication-assisted treatment, harms reduction approaches, and abstinence-based programs, which include Alcoholics Anonymous (AA) and other Twelve-Step Facilitation (TSF) approaches. There has been no consensus on the best way to treat AUD, and the most recent research affirms that there is no one-size-fits-all approach to recovery (Kelly, Humphreys, & Ferri, 2020; Kelly & Hoeppner, 2013; Lopez, 2020).

Likewise, while certainly not the only means to recovery, AA is one of the oldest and most well-known approaches to maintaining abstinence from alcohol. It is estimated that 70% of treatment facilities in the United States use AA/TSF treatment approaches and methods (Glaser, 2015). In a 2019 metadata analysis of 27 relevant studies, including over 10,000 participants, John Kelly,

DOI: 10.4324/9781003144854-8

Keith Humphreys, and Marcia Ferri (2020) found that "manualized AA/TSF interventions are more effective than other established treatments," and even nonmanualized AA/TSF "may perform as well as these other established treatments." Moreover, because it is available worldwide, free of charge, it is, as addiction specialist Kelly noted "the closest thing to a free lunch in public health" (Dossett, 2017, p. 942). Therefore, improving AA for all people—even while recognizing and developing alternatives—is important.

Despite its success and its other appealing attributes, though, AA remains a somewhat controversial approach to the treatment of alcoholism.[1] Groups like "SMART Recovery," Stanton Peele's "Life Process Program," and "LifeRing" all emerged as alternatives to AA. Additionally, the androcentrism of AA led to groups centered specifically on the unique challenges faced by women. Programs like "Tempest," the recovery approach founded by Holly Whitaker, author of *Quit Like a Woman*; Stephanie Covington's "trauma-informed and gender-sensitive programs"; and "Women for Sobriety" created mutual support networks that are replacements for AA. Researchers have compared these programs in terms of approaches and effectiveness (Tsutsumi, Timko, & Zemore, 2020; Zemore et al., 2017); the main relevant finding for the current chapter is that mutual-help groups can provide safe environments conducive to recovery for women, yet AA still needs to be responsive to its engagement with women as AA remains the most widely known, accessible, and free option for AUD treatment. As Christine Timko (2008) observed, too, AA's "ideological flexibility" allows it to appeal to a wide variety of special populations—including women.

We hope to contribute to the continuing conversations on recovery from AUD, women, and AA. It is estimated that 38% of AA members are women (AA, 2014). Previous research on women's participation in AA has, like this chapter, noted the importance of examining women's lived experience and narrative expression of that experience. Rachel Kornfield (2014) noted, for example, "the centrality of storytelling in constructing an alcoholic identity," which makes it "important to consider how AA's narrative structure can or cannot accommodate such [women's lived] experiences[2]" (417). Indeed, women do have experiences with AUD that are often distinct from men's experiences. The National Institute on Drug Abuse reported, for instance, that physical and sexual trauma "seem to be more common in substance-abusing women than in men," making the inclusion of such experiences in narrative form potentially helpful for women in recovery (Summary: Substance use in women research report, 2020). Recognizing that physical and sexual trauma as unifying experiences aren't the only attributes that make women's experiences unique, we argue that narrative-based approaches in AA need to be inclusive of all women+. In this chapter, thus, we provide a brief overview of AA with specific emphasis on the place of women. Our objective is to intervene in the hegemony of the book *Alcoholics Anonymous: The Story of How Many Thousands of Men and Women*

Have Recovered from Alcoholism in ways that call attention to the narrow representation of women and the constraints placed on what a woman is, or could be, according to the stories offered.

History and Background of Alcoholics Anonymous

AA was started in 1935 by Bill Wilson and Dr. Bob Smith. An abstinence-based program of recovery, AA has helped millions of people recover from alcoholism in an ever-growing worldwide fellowship. The core of the AA program encourages individuals to admit their powerlessness over alcohol, identify their character defects, and direct their attention to the "constant thought of others" in carrying the message of recovery (*Alcoholics Anonymous*, p. 20). As a result of adherence to the program, individuals "have recovered from a seemingly hopeless state of mind and body" and are able to be productive members of society once again (*Alcoholics Anonymous,* p. xiii).

The rhetorical construction of what it means to be "recovered" and the essential role of narrative is articulated through the foundational text, *Alcoholics Anonymous,* fondly referred to by members as "The Big Book." The forward to the second edition cites Dr. Bob Smith's recovery as proof that "one alcoholic could affect another as no nonalcoholic could" (p. xvi). Narrative is recognized as central to the transmission of the solution as it contributes to a person's sense of who they've been and who they can become, and "until such an understanding is reached, little or nothing can be accomplished" (*Alcoholics Anonymous,* p. 18). Additionally, the ability of potential alcoholics to see themselves in those who have recovered is integral to the personal commitment to AA and recovery.

The centrality of narrative as the means to recovery is evidenced in several ways within AA. The Big Book notes, "Our stories disclose in a general way what we used to be like, what happened, and what we are like now" (p. 58); this well-known excerpt from the chapter titled "How it Works" is read at the start of many meetings and functions to describe the narrative arc adhered to by the personal stories in the book, speakers at speaker meetings, and, more generally, at discussion-based meetings. Narrative provides the primary means by which potential adherents of the program identify with other members, orient themselves to the program of recovery, and describe who they are as a result of participation in AA. Furthermore, narrative is used to illustrate each of the key principles within the book *Alcoholics Anonymous.* For example, in the chapter, "More About Alcoholism," potential members of AA learn "to determine, to their own satisfaction" whether they belong in AA via four narrative examples that "describe some of the mental states that precede a relapse into drinking" (pp. 34–35). Here, the physical and emotional symptoms are constructed through personal stories rather than medical or psychological description or discussion. More crucial to the current analysis still is the space dedicated in each edition to personal stories of members.[3] Since each successive iteration dedicates more and more pages to include first-person narratives, *Alcoholics Anonymous* indicates the importance of narrative to identification as an alcoholic as well as it reinforces consistent elements and attitudes that persist across narratives of success.

While the first 164 pages of The Big Book have become sacred and remain unchanged, our intervention in the form of a call for more inclusivity is justified by cofounder Bill Wilson (1949), who wrote, "God forbid that Alcoholics Anonymous ever become frozen or rigid in its ways of doing or thinking. Within the framework of our principles the ways are apparently legion" (*Letter from Bill W. to Ed W.*). It is our intention to demonstrate that the values, principles, behaviors, and attitudes that are promoted as beneficial to successful recovery are narrowly conscripted onto "woman" and need to be negotiated by individuals trying to recover in AA.[4] Our narrative focus is particularly important since identification of "one alcoholic to another" is what "plants the seed" of hope that recovery is possible.[5] Additionally, as recognized by Kathy Lay and Susan G. Larimer (2018), there is a need to "appreciate women's experiences and their voices in recovery" (p. 635).

For this analysis, we establish Evelyn Brooks Higginbotham's (1994) idea of "respectability politics" as a useful frame within which to examine the rhetoric surrounding "the woman problem" as well as the recovery stories told by women. Attention to the narrative parameters of what is included by women when they share "what we used to be like.... And what we are like now" (*Alcoholics Anonymous,* p. 58) exposes how the rhetorical constraints of respectability *articulated by women* influence other women attempting recovery. Our rhetorical analysis is organized into three main sites of tension: the narrative defining of what it means to be "a lady,"[6] the normalization of heteronormativity and prioritization of family over self, and the way socioeconomic class is woven into the fabric of "acceptable woman." Within each of these sites of tension, we toggle back and forth between the tropes: "what we were like" and "what we are like now" to expose the standards women are asked to live up to and the narratives that are offered as metrics by which women should measure themselves.

History of Women in AA

Many sources have acknowledged that AA was primarily created by men, for men (McClellan, 2017; Schaberg 2019; Whitaker, 2019). As Holly Whitaker (2019) noted, it is important to remember "who [AA] was formed for, and why the program worked for its members," specifically, "upper-middle class white Protestant men in 1930s America ..." (p. 109). Michelle L. McClellan (2017) extended the observation to recognize the consequence to women and remarked that the "fellowship" of AA is like a fraternity, with its attendant traditions, rituals, and values that make it all the more difficult for women to become members. Likewise, John F. Kelly and Bettina B. Hoeppner's 2013 study established that men and women have "differing needs based on recovery challenges related to gender-based social roles and drinking contexts" (p. 186).

Thus, based on how AA was created and whom it was designed to serve, the early experiences of women in AA were challenging and complicated. Women had to overcome dual challenges: contending with societal attitudes that "good" women could not be alcoholics, and, based on this belief, being unwelcome at meetings during the initial years of AA (Schaberg, 2019). Mc-Clellan (2017) noted that "alcoholism, generally considered a man's disease, marked female sufferers as different, unusual, even 'unnatural' among those who manifested the condition ..." (p. 20). Even Sister Ignatia, quoted in *Dr. Bob and the good oldtimers* (1980), a pioneer in developing alcoholic treatment centers, "found it difficult to understand how a 'nice' girl could have a drinking problem" (p. 245). William H. Schaberg (2019) described "the woman alcoholic ... as a disreputable fallen creature who was unlikely to ever regain her former reputation" (p. 348). The negative stigma associated with women who drank was therefore reinforced nearly universally, and women seeking recovery needed to admit their alcoholism with all its attendant behavior and consequences while somehow also remaining a lady.

This way of thinking followed women into the rooms of AA, where one of the founders, Dr. Bob, was unsure if women could even find recovery in AA. He "showed somewhat less assurance upon confronting the most troublesome and, in some ways the most unwelcome minority in AA's olden days—women!" (*Dr. Bob and the Good Oldtimers*, 1980, p. 241).[7] This reluctance to accept women was confounded by the fact that the first women involved with AA were the wives of alcoholics. Their role was to be helpmates in maintaining their husband's sobriety. This characterization is exemplified in Chapter Eight of the Big Book, which was written "To Wives" and penned by one of the cofounders of AA, Bill Wilson,[8] despite Wilson's wife, Lois, offering to write the chapter. Additionally, the distinction made between wives and women alcoholics divided women affected by a common disease.[9]

To complicate things further, female alcoholics were often viewed as sexually loose women and a threat to the sobriety of the men in the program. According to Schaberg (2019), "Every woman who came in alone was like a warning signal to all the wives. They were scared to death of them" (p. 348). An early saying in AA, "under every skirt there's a slip," perfectly encapsulated one of the major challenges female alcoholics faced being accepted into the program by not only male alcoholics but also their wives.[10]

This positioning of women as problematic within the "halls" of AA was most completely articulated by an article appearing in the 1946 *Grapevine*,[11] written by Grace O. titled "Women in AA Face Special Problems," which was prominently displayed on the front page of the newsletter, and the article continued throughout several pages. Under the subheading, "Female Frailties," she wrote:

1 The percentage of women who stay in AA is low. Too many of them drop out after the novelty wears off...
2 Many women form attachments too intense—bordering on the emotional. Best-friends, crushes, hero-worship cause strained relationships.
3 So many women want to run things. To boss, manage, supervise, regulate, and change things...
4 Too many women don't like women.
5 Women talk too much. Gossip is a cancer to all AA groups and must be constantly watched. Men gossip far too much, too. But few use it for punishment, or revenge, or cutting someone down to size. ... [W]omen worry the same dead mouse until it's unrecognizable.
6 Women are a questionable help working with men and vice versa...
7 Sooner or later, a woman-on-the-make sallies into a group, on the prowl for phone numbers and dates...
8 A lot of women are attention-demanders and Spotlight sisters. They want to be spoonfed [sic], coaxed, babied, encouraged, teased, praised and personally conducted into sobriety.
9 Few women can think in the abstract. Everything must be taken personally. Universal truths to many women, are meaningless generalities. These women are impatient of philosophy, meditation and discussion...
10 Women's feelings get hurt too often...
11 Far too many women AAs cannot get along with the non-alcoholic wives of AA members. They feel ashamed or defiant, and they show it (Grace O., 1946, p. 1).

This list of "facts" identifies supposed "inherent" female characteristics that must be addressed for women alcoholics to be deemed respectable and, thereby, earn membership in an organization whose only "requirement for membership is an honest desire to stop drinking" (*Alcoholics Anonymous,* p. xiv). The subtext of the list makes it clear that a woman's respectability is always suspect and that participation in AA requires respectability. Theoretically, then, respectability politics (Higginbotham, 1994) serves as the foundation of our analysis to understand how the notion of "woman" as an alcoholic was problematized specifically through the promotion of being a "lady," highlighting the imperative for women in AA to behave in certain ways to attain successful recovery from alcoholism via the program.

Respectability Politics

Evelyn Higginbotham (1994) argued that certain behaviors are expected from nondominant members of society if they are to gain respect from dominant members. Known as Respectability Politics (aka Politics of Respectability), Higginbotham, in her study of Black women in the Black Baptist church, asserted that nondominant members held each other accountable based on cultural expectations of what a respectable person looks and acts like. Higginbotham stated that the "[t]he Baptist's women's emphasis on respectable behavior contested the plethora of negative stereotypes by introducing alternate images of Black women" (p. 191). These expectations relied on "… the visible assimilation of the dominant society's sexual codes and other 'ladylike' behavior" (p. 204).

While Higginbotham's work is used primarily to understand and critique the hegemonic cultural constraints placed on Black women, it has also been applied to same-sex marriage (Mastick & Conley, 2015), religious freedom (Miller & Towns, 2019), Latina behavior in politics and popular culture (Matos, 2019), and social class and digital self-presentation (Pitcan, Marwick, & Boyd, 2018). We argue that Respectability Politics provides a theoretical framework through which we might gain a better understanding of how women in AA sought/seek to conform themselves to the politics of grace and dignity—having to meet the challenge of not only being able to identify oneself as an alcoholic but to then also be seen as worthy of membership into a program that can and does save lives.

Analysis

Before exploring the three specific sites of tension central to the definition of a woman in AA, we need to point out the structural factors at work in the selection and arrangement of the stories section in the book *Alcoholics Anonymous* (1939, 1955, 1976, 2001). The current analysis draws on only the first two editions, arguing that it is in these early inclusions where we see the establishment of the parameters of what it means to be a woman in AA—limitations that remain in place in later editions.

Table 5.1 shows where each story we analyze can be found.

The first edition included only two stories by women—"A Feminine Victory" by Florence Rankin and "An Alcoholic's Wife" by Marie Bray.[12] Additionally, we draw from the story "My Wife and I" as someone perusing the story titles may be more likely drawn to this as it explicitly includes women, and as it directly describes gendered roles, even though it is not the story of a woman as told by a woman. The second edition included 11 stories by women. In this edition, stories were categorized into one of three types: "Pioneers," "They Stopped in Time," and "They Lost Nearly All." "Pioneers" included stories by the first people to coalesce around the name AA. "They Stopped in Time" included stories from members who did not hit as dramatic a "rock bottom" as those in "They Lost Nearly All." Despite our choice to focus on narratives in the first two editions, we do observe the changes made in the later editions with an eye to gender, yet we note the ways they nonetheless continue

TABLE 5.1 Personal Stories from *AA*

Story Title	First Appearance	Last Appearance
"A Feminine Victory"	1st Edition	1st Edition
"My Wife and I"	1st Edition	1st Edition
"An Alcoholics Wife"	1st Edition	1st Edition
"Women Suffer Too"	2nd Edition	*still included*
"From Farm to City"	2nd Edition	3rd Edition
"The Keys of the Kingdom"	2nd Edition	*still included*
"Fear of Fear"	2nd Edition	*still included*
"A Flower of the South"	2nd Edition	3rd Edition
"The Housewife who Drank at Home"	2nd Edition	*still included*
"Stars Don't Fall"	2nd Edition	3rd Edition
"Promoted to Chronic"	2nd Edition	3rd Edition
"Annie the Cop Fighter"	2nd Edition	2nd Edition
"The Independent Blonde"	2nd Edition	2nd Edition
"Freedom from Bondage"	2nd Edition	*still included*

the trajectories set out for women in the early editions. These categories are maintained in subsequent editions, and the distribution of stories by women in later versions supports our argument that AA presents a certain conception of women. For example, between the second and fourth editions, women become more likely to end up in the section "They Stopped in Time." Likewise, while the number of women included in "They Lost Nearly All" did increase with each edition, this section was also the space in which a Native American woman and a Black woman were included. This is not to say that there are not minority women who indeed have "Lost Nearly All," but to not recognize that there are also many who "Stopped in Time," and to present minority women as "last-gaspers" marks them with stigma. The inclusion of minority women in this section is also problematic in that, while these stories are inspirational, they also tokenize, and therefore, distance minority women from the larger communities of both AA and women in AA. Overall, the narratives selected for inclusion have consistently been from white, heteronormative women of privilege, and even as subsequent editions have included more voices, success for women has been defined by their ability to adopt and perform those values put forward in the early editions and perpetuated in tacit ways in later editions. Below, we share our analyses to further substantiate this point.

Women Drinkers

In The Big Book, the category of woman is problematized not only through the structural selection and inclusion of particular stories but also through the rhetorical construction of what it means to be a woman. In particular, a clear message on what it means to be a "lady" is infused throughout the pages of *Alcoholics Anonymous.* Gendered standards of behavior, of appropriate thoughts, and of desires are described throughout the text.[13] According to The Big Book, the female alcoholic had a particularly tough road to navigate in that she needed to remain a lady, but was compelled by alcohol to do "absurd, incredible, tragic things while drinking" (*AA,* p. 21).[14] The rhetoric used to describe drinking women functions to position it as "incredible" and out of the ordinary. Furthermore, the book makes it clear that women do unbecoming things *while drinking*, thereby implying that the cessation of drinking will correct any deviance. Women alcoholics explicitly recognized the difficulty in regaining their lost status as "ladies" in their narratives. The first sentence of "A Feminine Victory," for example, acknowledges Rankin had the "doubtful distinction of being the only 'lady' alcoholic in our particular section" (p. 216). Likewise, "Fear of Fear," one of the five stories from the early editions that remains in the most recent fourth edition, previews the story with "This lady was cautious" (p. 321).

Alcoholic women also indicate their appropriateness by identifying particular reasons for their drinking that are consistent with being a lady. For example, "A Feminine Victory" describes how the narrator got her first drink from her husband—she "had never known anything about it until I was almost thirty years old and he [husband] gave me my first drink" (p. 219). Also acceptable at the time was to use alcohol medicinally. "A Housewife Who Drank at Home," for instance, attributes "a period of particular stress and strain" for the use of alcohol "as a means of temporary release, as a means of getting a little extra sleep" (p. 235). Likewise, in "A Flower of the South" the narrator describes being "in a terrific state" on her wedding day when her father "taking things in hand" had a servant fetch some bourbon. She reflects that "it was really medicinal that night" but later "something went haywire" (p. 368). Medicinal use of alcohol is highlighted as a way of dealing with stress or trauma, making the eventual decline into alcoholism more understandable and appropriate. Additionally, the proffering of alcohol by a male authority figure further sanctions women's drinking. These women are not drinking for selfish reasons; rather they are drinking to perform their roles appropriately.

Women storytellers also position their drinking as the cause of their deviance from ladylike behavior and respectability. For example, in "From Farm to City," the narrator describes drinking more and more and, as a result, becoming "more defiant toward everything and everybody" (p. 264). Relatedly, when describing what they were like, narrators often distance themselves from popular tropes associated with alcoholics. For example, in "Fear of Fear" the author writes, "I never went to a hospital. I never lost a job. I was never in jail. And, unlike many others, I never took a drink in the morning" (p. 323). Thus, she describes her alcoholism as individualized, separating her from the larger category of women. Deviance from respectability is also individualized, which separates the alcoholic woman from "normal" women. In "Women Suffer Too," for example, the author describes her ordinariness: "The year after coming out, I married. So far, so good—all according to plan, like thousands of others" but, then notes, "But then the story became my own" (p. 225). In individualizing their alcoholism, women alcoholic storytellers reinforce stigma associated with harmful drinking and women—despite the acknowledgement that alcoholism is a disease.

Family First

The second site of tension where women had to navigate their performance of alcoholism revolved around the normalization of heteronormativity and prioritization of family over self.[15] Throughout the pages of *Alcoholics Anonymous*, it is repeated over and over that the individual who is a "real" alcoholic is powerless over alcohol. Despite the best intentions, alcoholics—"subjects of King Alcohol, shivering denizens of his mad realm"—are unable to meet their obligations and often act contrary to their moral principles (p. 151). In "Stars Don't Fall," the narrator describes her drinking: "I knew in my heart that I was unfit for the very things I wanted most, a happy marriage, security, a home, and love" (p. 403). So despite her alcoholism and active drinking, she maintains appropriate values and desires, and her deviance in behavior can be excused.

Despite the centrality of powerlessness as a precursor to recovery, women describe how the power of a mother's role can exert positive influence over the progression of their disease and subsequent recovery in their stories. For example, in "Fear of Fear," the narrator describes, "We had a small child, and I loved her dearly, so that held me back quite a bit in my drinking career" (p. 322). By using family—especially children—as a mitigating factor in their alcoholism, women present motherhood as a powerful force, and because they are affected by it (often through guilt and shame), they affirm their appropriateness in adhering to that role. In this way, they reinforce what Michelle McClellan (2017) identified as a general cultural perception of women's drinking as dangerous to "family stability and social harmony" (p. 6).

The prioritization of family is most evident in these narratives when women describe "what they are like now" in that most women center the benefits of sobriety, and their return to normalcy, around the family. When listing the benefits of surrendering to her disease, for instance, "The Housewife Who Drank at Home" lists "the ability to run my home, to face my responsibilities as they should be faced, to take life as it comes ..." (p. 340). Interestingly, several women writing in the early editions, when describing their sober lives switch from an "I" perspective to one which includes their husband, "we." For example, in "From Farm to City," the narrator notes "We [she and her husband] were in AA three and a half years" and "I always feel that our God consciousness was a steady growth after we became associated with AA. And we loved every minute of that association" (p. 270). Not only does this admission reinforce the narrator's behavior as aberrant from "normal women," but it also allows her to reassert and return to the mantle of wife. As a recovered wife, her feelings and actions are in line, and indeed indistinguishable, from those of her husband. Being recovered, then, means assuming the appropriate role of mother and wife.

Ladies Again

The final identity category significant to the establishment of respectability for the woman alcoholic is socioeconomic class. In the first two editions, several of the 12 stories by female alcoholics establish their position as respectable, appropriately stationed women. Among these women, they "attended the best boarding schools" ("Women Suffer Too", p. 225), were "given every advantage in a well-ordered home" ("Keys of the Kingdom", p. 304), and were introduced to alcohol through "cocktail parties, dances and night spots" ("A Flower of the South", p. 384). In "Stars Don't Fall" the "titled lady" reports being born "in a castle—the family home" where she lived "with servants and all the luxuries that I could possibly ask for" (pp. 400–401). The extreme wealth put on display through these stories, of course, limits the number of women who can relate to them and ignores the socioeconomic conditions that affect many other female alcoholics. The insinuation is, of course, that poor women are not a fit for AA.

Likewise, recovery from alcoholism for women is presented as a reinstatement of status—or an achievement of status previously unavailable. In "Annie The Cop Fighter," the narrator describes a "low bottom" in that she lost her husband and sons, lived without them for years, and was incarcerated several times for, as the title intimates, fighting with the police. Her life with her husband and children she describes as "too much of a decent life for me to lead" (p. 517). She goes on to describe how, on Mother's Day, she called her friend Irene from AA and "sobered up that very night after thirty-two years of knocking liquor around" (p. 519). Following a relapse eight months later—which is attributed to her lack of integration into the AA community—she returns "a new woman" (p. 520). She credits AA with giving her back her "respect" and "the love of everybody," she knows and credits AA with teaching her to be "humble" when she has "to be humble" (p. 522). Respect and humility are arguably synonyms for "dignity and grace." Dignity signifies the self-respect, self-control, and restraint necessary for women to possess and exert over themselves—and implicitly their sexual conduct. Grace implies a more public performance of femininity. Graceful women are humble, quiet, and effortlessly able to maintain their emotional nature while executing their duties as wife and mother.

Socioeconomic class status, however, is interestingly positioned as secondary to broader gender expectations about appropriate female behavior.

Interestingly, in the story "Stars Don't Fall," the author implies that despite being born into extreme wealth, when she loses the favor of her family, she reports: "I moved into a small apartment where I learned to cook, keep house, and do the things that normal people do. I learned a whole new sense of values" (p. 409). Acquiring the skills of home management earns her virtue within the pages of *Alcoholics Anonymous* and among AA members. Her road to recovery results in her recognition: "I am no longer interested in living in a palace, because palace living was not the answer for me" (p. 416). Instead, she reports that by taking the actions suggested by AA "going to meetings and listening, occasionally speaking, through doing Twelve Step work" she has "been taught all the things in life that are worth having" (p. 416). Repeatedly, the narratives in *Alcoholics Anonymous* highlight the virtues of femininity as sufficient for success, which obfuscates the very real obstacles that affect women not born into wealth.

Conclusion

It is important to expose the characterizations of "alcoholic women" and "recovered women" as described by AA since it is a "fellowship" that highlights the importance of identification of "one alcoholic with another." As demonstrated in this analysis, the conception of women described in the early literature sanctioned by AA is narrow and very much entrenched in whiteness, heteronormativity, and class status. In their stories, women are positioned as appropriate by positioning their drinking as unique to themselves, thereby keeping other women safe from the stigma and threat that they could fall victim to "King Alcohol." They drink because of stress or to get more sleep—in short, because they could not navigate their responsibilities as wives and mothers appropriately. Furthermore, their drinking is the cause of their deviance from suitable behavior. It is because of alcohol that they become argumentative, selfish, or unproductive.

Structurally, an intervention regarding the quality of stories included in the book *Alcoholics Anonymous* could ensure more inclusive representation of all people and circumstances, which could create a text that is welcoming and familiar for all of those who struggle with alcohol dependence, lessening the work that women need to do to see themselves in the pages of the basic text of *Alcoholics Anonymous*.[16] Rhetorical interventions in AA include spotlighting women+'s lived experience with alcoholism and normalizing their roads to recovery. Additionally, broadening the shared history of the creation of AA to recognize the work of women in creating and shaping the program would work to value women—both alcoholic and nonalcoholic—and the significant contributions they have made. While "there exists strong sentiment against any radical changes being made in it [the Big Book]" (p. xi, 4th edition), our hope is that the inclusion of all members is not considered "radical."

Because identification is crucial to the AA model of recovery, including more voices and more experiences in the narratives of "What we were like, what happened, and what we are like now" could make the book richer and more inclusive, welcoming more people who could think, "Yes, I am one of them, too; I must have this thing" (*Alcoholics Anonymous*, p. 29). Removing antiquated gender stereotypes and distributing women+ in the various sections mindfully should be front and center as the General Service Conference considers the adoption of a fifth edition of *Alcoholics Anonymous*. AA is a recovery program that has saved millions. However, that does not mean it, too, like its members, doesn't have "room to grow."

Notes

1 Books like Joe Miller's (2019) *US of AA: How the Twelve Steps Hijacked the Science of Alcoholism*, and Dodes and Dodes (2014) *The Sober Truth: Debunking the Bad Science Behind 12-Step Programs and the Rehab Industry*, critique approaches to AUD, especially in the U.S.
2 Kornfield's study informs ours, but diverges in that she studies a group of women who came together in a "Circle of Women" to provide support deliberately outside of AA.
3 The "basic text" of the Big Book, which describes how AA works to address alcoholism, spans 186 pages (including prefaces, forwards to older editions, and The Doctor's Opinion), in contrast to the 388 pages in the 4th edition that contain the stories of AA members.
4 In our next project, we plan to collect narratives describing the lived experiences of women+ trying to recover in AA. The current essay, however, articulates the reality created through the canonical text of the Big Book to understand the standards against which women+ are expected to measure themselves and their progress in recovery.
5 The centrality of narrative to AA has been noted by several sources (Ermann, 2013; Kornfield, 2014; Lay & Larimer, 2018). Not only are there stories in the back of each edition which members are encouraged to consult and "identity with," but each of the main principles or observations within the text are supported with personal examples – exclusively from men.
6 The assumption of whiteness associated with being a "lady" has been well documented (see Dyer, 2017).
7 Anecdotally, we can say that despite Dr. Bob's protestations, other early literature – and even early stories by women included in the Big Book – describe the wives of those in recovery as helpful to women trying to recover in AA. This dissonance – between what men say and what women experience – is not unique to AA, nor is it limited to this early phase of AA's history.
8 Interestingly, Lorrayne Carroll's (2007) concept of *rhetorical drag* is operational here in that Wilson, when writing "To Wives," wrote in the first person claiming, "As wives of AA, we would like you to feel that we understand as perhaps few can" (p. 104). The chapter then goes on to recount, in exacting detail, what a wife may feel and how she should respond to her alcoholic husband.
9 Al-Anon Family Groups, founded in 1951, eventually became a separate "program" designed for those affected by someone else's alcoholism. As with all 12-step programs the focus of Al-Anon is on the individual participant, not on the individual with alcoholism.

10 Even more daunting were the challenges faced by Women of Color (WOC), who not only bore the burden of being female, but faced the challenge of dealing with racist stereotypes in addition to having to create their own AA meetings amid segregation in the U.S. While outside the scope of the current analysis, Women of Color, and the additional labor necessary for them to fit into AA has received some academic attention (for example, see Kornfield, 2014) but obviously, there is more work to be done.

11 *Grapevine* is the international journal of AA, often called their "meeting in print."

12 It should be noted, however, that names were not—nor are they currently— included with stories. Instead, stories are known only by their title.

13 While outside the scope of the current paper, the text of the first 164 pages – the "sacred" pages which remain unchanged in each subsequent edition, describe the proper sphere of women primarily as wife. Even the chapter "To Wives" acknowl- edges "With few exceptions, our book thus far has spoken of men. But what we have said applies quite as much to women. Our activities in behalf of women who drink are on the increase." But it then goes on to dedicate the entire chapter to the "wife who trembles in fear" (p. 104) and explains the behavior of the husband and how the wife can be most useful.

14 As noted by Kathy Lay and Susan Larimer (2018), scholars have recognized the centrality of trauma as a "crucial part of women's recovery programs (Harris et al., 2005; Linton et al., 2009)" (p. 626). The experience of trauma, and the integration of trauma into the healing process is noticeably absent from the stories included in the Big Book.

15 Identification of these values also begs the question raised by Michelle McClellan (2017) who recognizes the larger issue of "the failure of treatment regimes to accommodate alcoholic women's domestic obligations and lack of power in the family" (p. 3).

16 As evidenced by the plethora of recovery programs emerging over the last 20 years, people will find ways to recover outside of AA. It is also not our intention to suggest that *AA* is the only way—or even the best way—to recovery. We do, however, hope that this analysis can suggest some paths forward for AA.

References

AA. (2014). "2014 Membership Survey." *aa.org.*

Alcoholics Anonymous. (1980). *Dr. Bob and the good oldtimers: A biography, with recollec- tions of early A.A. in the Midwest.* AA World Services, Inc.

Alcoholics Anonymous: The story of how thousands of men and women have recovered from alco- holism (1st ed.). (1939). AA World Services, Inc.

Alcoholics Anonymous: The story of how thousands of men and women have recovered from alco- holism (2nd ed.). (1955). AA World Services, Inc.

Alcoholics Anonymous: The story of how thousands of men and women have recovered from alco- holism (3rd ed.). (1976). AA World Services, Inc.

Alcoholics Anonymous: The story of how thousands of men and women have recovered from alco- holism (4th ed.). (2001). AA World Services, Inc.

Carroll, Lorrayne. (2007). *Rhetorical drag: Gender impersonation, captivity, and the writing of history.* The Kent State University Press.

Dossett, Wendy. (2017). A daily reprieve contingent on the maintenance of our spiri- tual condition. *Addiction, 112*(6), 924–943.

Dyer, Richard. (2017). *White: Twentieth anniversary edition.* Routledge.

Ermann, Lauren Sheli. (2013). The lived experiences of older women in AA. (Publication No. 146885155) [Doctoral Dissertation, Virginia Polytechnic Institute]. Semantic Scholar.

Glaser, Gabrielle. (2015). *The irrationality of AA*. The Atlantic. https://www.theatlantic.com/magazine/archive/2015/04/the-irrationality-of-alcoholics-anonymous/386255/

Grace, O. (1946). Women in AA face special problems. *The AA Grapevine, III, 5,* 1–10.

Harris, M., Fallot, R., & Wolfson Berley, R. (2005). Qualitative interviews on substance abuse relapse and prevention among female trauma survivors. *Psychiatric Services, 56*(10), 1292–1296.

Higginbotham, Evelyn Brooks. (1994). *Righteous discontent: The women's movement in the Black Baptist church, 1880–1920.* Harvard University Press.

Kelly, John F., & Hoeppner, Bettina B. (2013). Does AA work differently for men and women? A moderated multiple-mediation analysis in a large clinical sample. *Drug and Alcohol Dependence, 130,* 186–193.

Kelly, John F., Humphreys, Keith, & Ferri, Marcia. (2020). AA and other 12-step programs for alcohol use disorder. *Cochrane Database of Systematic Reviews, 3,* doi:10.1002/14651858.CD012880.

Kornfield, Rachel. (2014). (Re)Working the program: Gender and openness in AA. *Ethos, 42*(4), 415–439.

Lay, Kathy, & Larimer, Susan G. (2018). Vigilance: The lived experience of women in recovery. *Qualitative Social Work, 17*(5), 624–638.

Linton, J., Flaim, M., Deulche C, et al. (2009). Women's experience in holistic chemical dependency treatment: An exploratory qualitative study. *Journal of Social Work Practice in the Addictions, 9*(3): 282–298.

Lopez, German. (2018, January 2). *Why some people swear by AA – and others despise it.* VOX. https://www.vox.com/policy-and-politics/2018/1/2/16181734/ 12-steps-aa-na-studies

Lopez, German. (2020, March 11). A new, big review of the evidence found that Alcoholics Anonymous works – for some. *VOX.* https://www.vox.com/science-and-health/2020/3/11/21171736/alcoholics-anonymous-cochrane-study-research

Matos, Amanda R. (2019). Alexandria Ocasio-Cortez and Cardi B. jump through hoops: Disrupting respectability politics when you are from the Bronx and wear hoops. *Harvard Kennedy School Journal of Hispanic Policy, 3,* 89–93.

Matsick, Jes L., & Conley, Terri D. (2015). Maybe "I do," maybe I don't: Respectability politics in the same sex marriage ruling. *Analyses of Social Issues and Public Policy, 15*(1), 409–413.

McClellan, Michelle L. (2017). *Lady lushes: Gender, alcoholism, and medicine in modern America.* Rutgers University Press.

Miller, Eric C., & Towns, James E. (2019). Religious freedom, respectability politics, and W.A. Criswell in 1960. *Rhetoric and Public Affairs, 22*(1), 33–57.

Murez, Cara. (2021, February 19). Drinking too much during the pandemic? *WebMD.* https://www.webmd.com/lung/news/20210219/drinking-too-much-during-the-pandemic#1

National Institute on Drug Abuse. (2020, May 27). Summary: Substance use in women research report. https://www.drugabuse.gov/publications/research-reports/substance-use-in-women/summaryr, 2021, from https://www.drugabuse.gov/publications/research-reports/substance-use-in-women/summary

National Institute on Drug Abuse. (2021, March.) *Alcohol facts and statistics.* https://www.niaaa.nih.gov/sites/default/files/publications/NIAAA_Alcohol_Facts_and_Stats_1.pdf

Pitcan, Mikaela, Marwick, Alice E., & boyd, danah. (2018). Performing a vanilla self: Respectability politics, social class, and the digital world. *Journal of Computer-Mediated Communication, 23,* 163–179.

Schaberg, William H. (2019). *Writing the big book: The creation of AA.* Central Recovery Press.

Timko, Christine. (2008). *Outcomes of AA for special populations.* VA Health Care System. https://www.mentalhealth.va.gov/providers/sud/selfhelp/docs/5_Outcomes_of_AA_for_Special_Populations.pdf

Tsutsumi, Shiori, Timko, Christine, & Zemore, Sarah. (2020). Ambivalent attendees: Transitions in group affiliation among those who choose 12-step alternatives for addiction. *Addictive Behaviors, 102,* 1–8.

Whitaker, Holly. (2019). *Quit like a woman: The radical choice to not drink in a culture obsessed with alcohol.* The Dial Press.

Wilson, Bill. (1949). *Letter from Bill W. to Ed W.* Harbor Area Central Organization of AA. https://hacoaa.org/documents/bill-w-to-ed-w/

Zemore, Sarah, Kaskautas, Lee Ann, Mericle, Amy, & Hemberg, Jordana. (2017). Comparison of 12-step groups to mutual help alternatives for AUD, a large national study: Differences in membership characteristics and group participation, cohesion, and satisfaction. *Journal of Substance Abuse Treatment, 73,* 16–26.

6

RHETORICAL CROCHETING

New Chinese Moms Fighting Postpartum Depression on Social Media

Hua Wang

Introduction

In the early morning of April 27th, 2020, a 37-year-old woman died by suicide in Changsha, China; she leapt off a high building to her death while holding her five-month-old daughter. It's reported that the deceased woman, Su, earned a PhD degree overseas, and the dead baby girl was her second child. After giving birth, Su developed symptoms of postpartum depression, but her family did not take her depression seriously. One of her family members, for instance, noted that they believed that her death was related to postpartum depression, yet, "didn't expect it to be so serious" (Cao, 2020). Due to her PhD degree, Su's death became a hashtag #37-year-old overseas female returnee with a PhD degree, with her 5-month-old daughter, jumped off the building to death# on Weibo, one of China's most popular social media sites. There were more than 1,600,000 clicks. The case fascinated the public. Many users did not understand how such a well-educated woman, with a good job and a happy family, could develop postpartum depression, and some users even said that higher education could not save her from postpartum depression (#37-year-old overseas female returnee with a PhD, with her 5-month-old daughter, jumped off the building to death#, 2020).

Their confusion revealed, of course, a shallow understanding of postpartum depression—a nonpsychotic depressive illness and one of the most common complications of the postpartum period. Postpartum depression is characterized by feelings of extreme sadness, anxiety, trouble sleeping, mood swings, and so on. It can last for weeks, months, or even more than a year; it can make it difficult for moms to take care of their newborn babies and themselves (Mayo Clinic). Research shows that 5–20% of mothers in high-income Western

DOI: 10.4324/9781003144854-9

countries and 25–36% in lower-income countries suffer from this maternal mental health problem (Ding et al., 2019). In China, postpartum depression is increasingly prevalent and ranks No. 2 after depression among China's top mental health problems. Additionally, in China, about 17% of new moms are diagnosed with severe postpartum depression, and up to 85% of moms may experience depressive feelings after giving birth (Ni, 2018).

The Chinese Weibo users' reaction to Su's death is not all that surprising. Postpartum depression is a new concept in Chinese culture, and the public knows little about it. Many Chinese people do not see postpartum depression as an illness, as in the case of Su who had symptoms but whose family did not pay attention to her depression. Depressed moms receive little support from their families (Ni, 2018). In addition, most Chinese people stigmatize postpartum depression. They regard tearfulness, fatigue, anxiety, and other symptoms of postpartum depression as signs of a new mom's weakness or her negative feelings. Many women feel ashamed to acknowledge that they have a mental disorder, and they are not likely to seek psychological consultation and medical treatment (Xu, 2019). Due to not getting consultations or medical treatment in a timely and appropriate manner, some depressed moms harm themselves and even die by suicide (Ni, 2018). The cases of depressed moms' self-harm and suicide are increasingly appearing in the Chinese media, which incorrectly signals that postpartum depression is inevitably self-destructive. The high-profile negative coverage of postpartum depression further stigmatizes postpartum depression, and many depressed moms feel sad and scared to admit that they have postpartum depression.

In China, the biased cultural discourse on postpartum depression silences sufferers and renders their pain invisible, which significantly impacts them and their families. This masking eventually leads to a collective unwillingness to accept postpartum depression as a mental disorder and to stigmatization against it. Therefore, a rhetorical response to cultural invisibility becomes essential.

In this chapter, I focus on a case study to scrutinize how a depressed Chinese new mom Mao Wan used the craft of crocheting to identify with other depressed moms on social media, and how they further identified with one another by sharing embodied experiences of postpartum depression. Through the embodied identification practice, they had a better understanding of the mental disorder and worked together to do a public crocheting artifact installation to raise the public's awareness of postpartum depression. I argue that the crocheting artifacts along with written signs in the installation work as material rhetoric, rhetorically intervening in the dominant narratives of postpartum depression in China.

After the overview of my methods and data collection, I provide a description of the frameworks of identification and material rhetoric. Then, I analyze how Mao Wan identified with other depressed moms by the craft of crocheting and sharing her embodied experiences. I also analyze how the women Mao

Wan networked with online worked together to use the crocheted artifacts as material rhetoric in a large-scale art installation designed to raise the public's awareness of and to destigmatize postpartum depression. I argue that the materiality of embodied experiences has the potential to intervene in the dominant narratives of mental health in communities such as China with strong stigmatization of mental disorders.

Methods and Data Collection

The case study in this chapter is focused on a Chinese new mom Mao Wan. She was a 30-year-old mother of two when she became an online celebrity in 2019 because of a video clip showing her handrail decorations of a shopping street in the Pudong New Area in Shanghai. Mao suffered postpartum depression after she gave birth to her first child in 2015. To divert her physical and mental discomfort, she picked up her hobby of crocheting, which eventually helped her recover from postpartum depression. She created three crocheting groups on social media totaling about 1,000 members, most of whom were young moms seeking to ease anxiety and pressure by crocheting. With the support of Jinxiu Fang, a property management company in charge of the shopping area, she and other moms from the crocheting groups spent months crocheting cute animals and ornate patterns to decorate the shopping street to mark World Mental Health Day on Oct 10, 2019. Chinese media covered Mao Wan's personal stories about fighting postpartum depression by crocheting as well as the colorful public art installation. This chapter draws on secondary sources in some influential news outlets in China, such as: *China Daily*, *The People's Daily*, *Xinjiang Daily*, Xinhuanet news portal, Sina news portal, and the Sohu news portal. I collected the following sources related to Mao Wan's online activism and public rhetoric project:

- The interviews of Mao Wan
- The coverages of Mao Wan's stories
- Seven images of her decorating the shopping street
- Ten images of cute crocheted animals sitting on the handrails of the shopping street
- Three images of the handrails decorated with colorful crocheted wipes
- Two images of the signs hung on the handrails
- One image of colorful crocheted umbrellas
- One image of colorful crocheted ice cream

These items make up an ideal corpus through which to highlight the rhetorical significance of Mao Wan and her activist project, which unexpectedly went viral on social media to raise more audiences' awareness. Mao Wan and her group's activist project did important work in bringing the plight of women suffering from postpartum depression to light since postpartum depression is stigmatized in China and most Chinese people lack awareness of it.

Theoretical Framework

Kenneth Burke (1969) developed the theory of identification that describes human interaction as not only for persuasion but also for a process of transformation and change in communication. He saw language as symbolic action to define the notion of rhetorical identification. He explained that "you persuade a man only insofar as you can talk his language by speech, gesture, tonality, order, images, attitude, idea, identifying your ways with his" (1969, p. 55). He also wrote that "non-verbal, situational factors" can participate in effective persuasion (p. 65). Hence, he suggested that rhetoricians do "the analysis of non-verbal factors wholly extrinsic to the rhetorical expression considered purely as a verbal structure" (p. 62). In this chapter, I blend this notion of identification with materiality and material rhetoric as they are used in other rhetoric of health and medicine (RHM) work such as in Maria Novotny's (2019) work where she and her collaborator Elizabeth Walker helped women create visual artifacts with narratives to express their embodied infertile experiences. Those visual stories implicitly serve as material rhetoric that may not only communicate painful experiences to viewers, making them identify with those who want to share the same stories, but also speak back to the dominant cultural narrative that assumes a female body is a fertile body and correlates womanhood with motherhood. In the same way, Mao Wan and her constituents use the craft of crocheting as a material rhetorical means to challenging the dominant and stigmatized cultural dispositions toward postpartum depression.

Material rhetoric adds an important layer to my analysis. Burke's identification does not fully enable an understanding of the necessity and the power of Mao Wan's story. Adding the material dimension moves Burke's identification into a new area that affords researchers better ways of understanding how people can shift their identities. In this case, it allows researchers to understand the impact of Mao Wan's story and the intercultural view of shifting the stigma of postpartum depression. The definition of "material rhetoric" was put forward by Michael McGee in the 1980s. He posited the idea that rhetoric should be viewed as material "because it survives and records the moment of experience" (qtd in Biesecker & Lucaites, 2009, p. 23). Many rhetorical scholars have followed his idea over the past several decades by recognizing the material impacts of rhetorical tactics and gradually moving the concept of material rhetoric toward social justice movements. For example, Richard Marback (1998) interpreted the closed fist in Detroit as powerful material rhetoric, designed to challenge racism. Similarly, Jamie White-Farnham (2013) identified the red and purple hats and costumes worn by members of a Rhode Island chapter of the Red Hat Society as material rhetoric to address the marginalization or invisibility of aging women. These examples powerfully demonstrate how material rhetoric inspires resistance to social norms and brings attention to marginalized groups.

Taken together, Burke's identification and material rhetoric offer a theoretical lens through which to interpret how Mao Wan identified with other new moms with postpartum depression on social media by means of the craft of crocheting and embodied personal experiences. This blending of Burke's identification with material rhetoric also helps to account for how women used their crocheted artifacts as individual statements that were part of the large-scale art installation meant to raise public awareness of postpartum depression. In this sense, the crocheted artifacts serve as material rhetoric that not only presents postpartum depression to the public but also intervenes in the dominant narratives of postpartum depression in China. The remainder of this chapter explains the rhetorical significance of Mao Wan and her activist project as it offered women space to externalize and symbolically recast the very real pain that they were in as they navigated postpartum depression.

Online activism, of course, is not new in China; it first appeared in the late 1990s (Yang, 2009). With the advancement of communication technologies, activists have recognized the potential of the Internet, especially social media, as a force for social change (Sutton & Pollock, 2000; Tai, 2015). Despite the government's sophisticated political control of online space, the past three decades in China have seen more frequent and influential online activities for various marginalized interests (Yang, 2009). For example, grassroots environmental activists use social media as a platform to share information, build social networking, mobilize the public, and construct a green public discourse (Sima, 2011; Sullivan & Xie, 2009). Because LGBT and feminist activism is strictly censored, social media is an important avenue for gender-related grassroots activists to present their voices and to put up collective resistance (Cao & Guo, 2016; Chase, 2012; Hou, 2015; Mao, 2020). Such that they might achieve the best outcome of their advocacy, feminist activists adopt various online strategies such as further politicizing women's private matters for provoking heated online discussion and building online coalitions to create spaces for women's voice (Hou, 2020; Wang & Driscoll, 2019). This chapter continues the scholarship on Chinese online activism via its engagement with Mao Wan's public campaign; it shows how the installation that she and her constituents created intervened in the dominant narratives of postpartum depression in China.

Using the Craft of Crocheting to Cope with Postpartum Depression and Identify with More Depressed Young Moms

According to the coverage of her story, Mao Wan's postpartum depression mirrors the experiences of other moms with postpartum depression around the globe, yet her experiences were also greatly related to Chinese sociocultural factors. In an interview with her from *Xinjiang Daily*, Mao Wan said that after the birth of her first child, she had difficulty accepting the scar from her C-section. The C-section incision pain and breastfeeding pain constantly bothered her. During her pregnancy, her family gave her substantial attention and care, but after childbirth, they shifted their focus to the newborn baby. She could not mentally adapt herself to the significant change in prenatal and postnatal attention. In addition, the traditional Chinese postpartum practices did not empower her to take on her role as a new mom. In the month after delivery, she was confined at her mother-in-law's home following strict dietary and behavioral restrictions. She was not allowed to eat vegetables, for example, or to open the windows or to turn on the air conditioning, though the weather was stuffy. She had not washed her hair in a month, which made her feel dirty and gloomy; she disliked herself. Moreover, she quit her job and stayed at home to take care of her baby, but she struggled in her new role as a mother. She felt useless and lost interest in life. She cried more than usual and could not sleep at night. She became reluctant to care for her baby and feared that she would do something harmful to him (Xu, 2019).

Like many other depressed young moms, postpartum depression stigma prevented Mao Wan from acknowledging that she was suffering from postpartum depression, and she refused to seek therapy. Instead, she picked up her hobby of crocheting to make some artifacts to combat her negative feelings (Xu, 2019). Thus, the craft of crocheting turned out to be an effective tool to help her cope with postpartum depression. In an interview, she said that when crocheting the artifacts, she concentrated on the crocheting skills and patterns and forgot the negative feelings. Gradually, she could sleep at night and had more energy to take care of her son (Xu, 2019). Mao Wan found that crocheting was therapeutic, and it helped to define goals: initially, to crochet a small hat and a few pairs of shoes for her baby. When she finished the hat, she took a picture of it and posted the picture on social media. Her friends' likes and praise helped to restore her self-confidence. As Mao Wan put it, "I posted the photo of the baby hat on social media, and it got me so much praise from my friends. I felt that I had finally done something valuable" (Shen, 2019). The sense of achievement that the craft of crocheting brought to her led her to create a social network account to share her achievements. Through crocheting and sharing, she gradually eliminated her negative feelings and constructed an identity as a confident new mother recovered from postpartum depression. She began interacting with her baby more positively by playing and talking with him, as she gradually accepted her new role as a mother (Shen, 2019). Since Mao Wan shared her crocheting skills and artifacts on social media, the craft of crocheting enacted a rhetorical function: it helped her to identify with her many followers who love crocheting and wanted to learn it—most of whom were also stay-at-home moms. She set up three groups on social media to teach them crocheting skills (Moms weave their way out of depression, 2019). Crocheting, in this way, worked as a means of identification by which the group members built a gendered virtual community where they constructed their new identities as traditional technique learners who were also engaged in a significant material process.

Mao Wan and her group members became further identified with one another by sharing their personal embodied experiences of reproduction and life. When teaching crocheting skills, Mao Wan told her group members that she had suffered from postpartum depression after childbirth and explained how the hobby of crocheting helped her recover from it. Meanwhile, the others shared their personal experiences about childbirth, parenting, and working. Mao Wan found that there were many moms with postpartum depression, and they either had not realized the illness or had refused to admit it due to the stigma attached to it. In an interview, Mao Wan explained,

> I not only share my crocheting skills, but also ask them about their working and living conditions and whether they have talked with their families (about their postpartum depression), and I suggest they go to visit a psychologist for serious symptoms.
>
> *(Moms weave their way out of depression, 2019)*

Gradually, some moms with light and mild postpartum depression symptoms eased their anxiety and depression symptoms by means of crocheting and eventually fought their way out of postpartum depression (He, 2019). This means of sharing embodied experiences became the key identification practice that helped the depressed moms acknowledge and assert their identity as individuals suffering from postpartum depression in the affirming social media community. This embodied identification practice improved understanding and prompted transformation and change among the group members. Moreover, the transformation and change that crocheting and sharing embodied experience brought to the social media community continues because Mao Wan said that she would explore ways to help the young moms turn their crocheting works into income, alleviating the stay-at-home moms' income pressure while creating a shared sense of accomplishment (He & Wang, 2019).

Using Crocheting Artifacts as Material Rhetoric to Combat the Dominant Narratives of Postpartum Depression

Apart from teaching crocheting in a social media community, Mao Wan did some research on crocheting and postpartum depression online. She found that in Western countries many crocheting lovers did large-scale art installations to raise public awareness of depressed patients, empty nest elderly, and autistic children. Mao Wan became inspired and wanted to do a similar public installation in China. Her intention was to alert Chinese society and families to the true nature of postpartum depression such that audiences might be moved to give more attention and care to the moms with postpartum depression, and, thus, help them recover from it. When she shared this destigmatizing idea with her group members, many of them applauded it. They decided to do a large-scale outdoor installation in the Jinxiufang shopping area (Wang & He, 2019). In thinking about the meaning of the installation, material rhetoric offers a fitting interpretative lens to examine the crocheted artifacts as they bring the public's attention to and raise awareness of postpartum depression.

To achieve their advocacy aim, Mao Wan and her group members took advantage of the public installation to express their perspective on postpartum depression. First, they used different colors of yarns to crochet 500 meters of colorful artifacts and more than 600 dolls and animals, decorating the iron handrails in the shopping area (Chen, 2019). The 24 images of the crocheted artifacts collected in the news outlets display some cute dolls, bears, angry birds, rabbits, ice creams, monkeys, and umbrellas. All of them were made in seven colors, which is called the rainbow[1] color, indicating that new moms should feel well enough to enjoy a good and happy mood. They also created signs with written words to educate the public and destigmatize postpartum depression. For example, the public installation included a sign with the words: "[w]e hope that our society can better understand postpartum depression and care more about it. Please face postpartum depression correctly and accompany her with love," indicating that postpartum depression is an illness, that society should not stigmatize it, and that families should give more attention and care to depressed moms (Fu, 2019).

Another two signs, one saying "[r]efuse to get depressed after childbirth and be a rainbow (happy) mom," (URL for location to follow at proof stage) and the other saying "Let's do crocheting together to make the unhappy mood gone stitch by stitch," (URL for location to follow at proof stage) seem aimed at educating women readers on how to cope with a depressed mood following childbirth (Chen, 2019; Fu, 2019).

These colorful crocheted artifacts considered in the framework of material rhetoric publicly "speak out" on what postpartum depression is; they bring postpartum depression visibility. They function as material activism in a deliberate and important way in that they attempt to change the public's perception of postpartum depression in a concrete way. As such, the colorful crocheted artifacts in the public installation serve as activism and function rhetorically in terms of providing women with an opportunity to mitigate stigma against postpartum depression so that women are better able to obtain family support and, when necessary, medical intervention.

Mao Wan's embodied postpartum depression experience helped make the public crocheting installation very successful and more new moms suffering from the illness came to join her (Moms weave their way out of depression, 2019). Mao Wan said in an interview,

Postpartum depression and depression have always been a serious topic. We hope that through this installation and our joint efforts, more and more people can pay attention to this topic, and patients will be able to recover as soon as possible.

(Wyrubywang, 2019)

These strong statements convey political and rhetorical significance. Though she said that she'd never expected that the outdoor installation would become a hot topic in the media, Mao Wan's embodied postpartum depression experiences as she shared them online and the offline outdoor installation invited a wider range of audiences to become aware of postpartum depression (Chen, 2019). Moreover, by means of social media, the subsequent actions that the crocheted artifacts installation induced furthered the transformation and change that happened beyond Mao Wan's crocheting social media community, moving forward to rhetorically respond to the dominant narratives of postpartum depression (He & Wang, 2019).

Conclusion and Implications

As cultural psychiatrists have long argued, any discourses on mental disorders must consider sociocultural factors. In China, mental disorders are deeply stigmatized and rendered invisible. Through the case of Mao Wan and other Chinese mothers coping with postpartum depression by crocheting, networking with other moms, and then using their crocheted artifacts in a public installation as material rhetoric to raise the public's awareness of postpartum depression, this chapter suggests that the materiality of personal embodied experience can be recast into material artifacts such that those suffering from mental health concerns can engage with and identify with audiences. When women come together to share their embodied experiences with postpartum depression and then work together to do this symbolic recasting work, it becomes possible to rhetorically intervene in dominant and stigmatizing mental health discourses in China. Mao Wan's feminist online activism not only contributes to the Chinese feminist movement, but it also echoes Western feminist scholars' work, especially in the field of RHM where breastfeeding women, pregnant teenagers, new moms, and infertile women employ their personal embodied experiences or stories as rhetorical interventions to combat dominant social, political, institutional, and cultural discourses (Koerber, 2006; Owens, 2015; Seigel, 2014; Vinson, 2018). The collective act of the crocheting in Mao Wan's case, thus, also highlights the role that social media plays in expanding the circulation of the Chinese moms' embodied experiences and stories of coping with postpartum depression. The large-scale installation used to raise the public's awareness came into being only after these moms connected and shared their experiences with each other online. This case, thus, reinforces the idea that social media is a potential tool to promote social justice. Meanwhile, this case aids in theorizing how reproductive injustice occurs in relation to institutional and cultural oppression in different cultures and groups, and how digital spaces are an ideal place for women to assert rhetorical agency in enacting intercultural communication of reproductive justice.

Note

1 In the US, rainbows are associated with healthy babies that are born following miscarriage(s) or infant loss.

References

Burke, Kenneth. (1969). *A grammar of motives*. University of California Press.

Cao, Wei. (2020, April 27). The 37-year-old female overseas returnee with a PhD degree, with her five-month daughter, committed suicide by jumping off the building. It's suspected that her death was due to postpartum depression (H. Wang, Trans.). *News Sina*. https://news.sina.com.cn/s/2020-04-27/doc-iirczymi8706381.shtml

Cao, Jin, & Guo, Lei. (2016). Chinese "Tongzhi" community, civil society, and online activism. *Communication and the Public*, *1*(4), 504–508.

Chase, Thomas. (2012). Problems of publicity: Online activism and discussion of same-sex sexuality in South Korea and China. *Asian Studies Review*, *36*(2), 151–170.

Chen, Sizhong. (2019, June 10). Fighting postpartum depression with wool yarns, this mother born in 90s is awesome! (H. Wang, Trans.). *Zhongxiang News*. https://baijiahao.baidu.com/s?id=1635949943248421386&wfr=spider&for=pc

Ding, Guodong, Niu, Lei, Binturache, Angela, Zhang, Jun, Lu, Min, Gao, Yu, Pan, Shuming, & Tian, Ying. (2019). "Doing the month" and postpartum depression among Chinese women: A Shanghai prospective cohort study. *Women and Birth*, *33*(2), 151–158.

Fu, Yang. (2019, April 20). The handrails of the streets in Pudong wearing colorful "sweaters", and the story behind it carried. *The People's Daily This Morning*! (H. Wang, Trans.). http://sh.eastday.com/m/20190420/u1ai12439156.html

He, Wenya. (2019, April 25). Why did she dress the entire street handrails in the "sweaters" that she crocheted? Young mom Mao Wan hopes to have more space to show the crochetwork from the group of crocheting lovers (H. Wang, Trans.). *Sina News*. https://finance.sina.com.cn/roll/2019-04-25/doc-ihvhiqax4885091.shtml

He, Xiyue, & Wang, Moling. (2019, October 10). Dressing sweaters for the streets: Chinese young mothers using crocheting to ease parenting anxiety (H. Wang, Trans.). *Sina News*. http://k.sina.com.cn/article_213815211_0cbe8fab02000pnmq.html

Hou, Holly Lixian. (2015). On fire in Weibo: Feminist online activism in China. *Economic and Political Weekly*, *50*(17), 79–85.

Hou, Holly Lixian. (2020). Rewriting "the personal is political": Young women's digital activism and new feminist politics in China. *Inter-Asia Cultural Studies*, *21*(3), 337–355.

Koerber, Amy. (2006). "Rhetorical agency, resistance, and the disciplinary rhetorics of breastfeeding". *Technical Communication Quarterly*, *15*, 87–101.

Mao, Chengting. (2020). Feminist activism via social media in China. *Asian Journal of Women's Studies, 26*(2), 245–258.

Marback, Richard. (1998). Detroit and the closed fist: Toward a theory of material rhetoric. *Rhetoric Review, 17*(1), 74–92.

Moms weave their way out of depression. (2019, October 22). *China Daily*. https://www.chinadaily.com.cn/a/201910/22/WS5dae6ebfa310cf3e35571df8_2.html

Ni, Dandan. (2018, July 12) The silent struggle of having postpartum depression in China. *Sixth Tone: Fresh Voices from Today's China*. https://www.sixthtone.com/news/1002609/the-silent-struggle-of-having-postpartum-depression-in-china

Novotny, Maria. (2019). The ART of infertility: Finding friendship & healing after reproductive loss. *Survive & Thrive: A Journal for Medical Humanities and Narrative as Medicine, 4*(1), 19.

Owens, Kim Hensley. (2015). *Writing childbirth: Women's rhetorical agency in labor and online*. Southern Illinois University Press.

Postpartum depression. Mayo Clinic. https://www.mayoclinic.org/diseases-conditions/postpartum-depression/symptoms-causes/syc-20376617

Seigel, Marika. (2014). *The rhetoric of pregnancy*. The University of Chicago Press.

Shen, Ke. (2019, October 11). Women are weaving their way out of postpartum depression (H. Wang, Trans.). *Shine News*. https://www.shine.cn/news/nation/1910113491/

Sima, Yangzi. (2011). Grassroots environmental activism and the Internet: Constructing a green public sphere in China. *Asian Studies Review, 35*(4), 477–497.

Sullivan, Jonathan, & Xie, Lei. (2009). Environmental activism, social networks and the internet. *The China Quarterly, 198*, 422–432. https://doi.org/10.1017/S0305741009000381

Sutton, Jo, & Pollock, Scarlet. (2000). Online activism for women's rights. *CyberPsychology & Behavior, 3*(5), 699–706.

Tai, Zixue. (2015). Networked resistance: Digital populism, online activism, and mass dissent in China. *Popular Communication, 13*(2), 120–131.

Vinson, Jenna. (2018). *Embodying the problem: The persuasive power of the teenage mother*. Rutgers University Press.

Wang, Bin, & Driscoll, Catherine. (2019). Chinese feminists on social media: Articulating different voices, building strategic alliances. *Continuum, 33*(1), 1–15.

Wang, Moling, & He, Xiyue, (2019, October 10) Shanghai "new mom" Mao Wan: Using wool crocheting to relieve anxiety (H. Wang, Trans.). *Sohu*. https://www.sohu.com/a/346083200_115402

White-Farnham, Jamie. (2013). Changing perceptions, changing conditions: The material rhetoric of the Red Hat Society. *Rhetoric Review, 32*(4), 473–489.

Wyrubywang. (2019, April 22). The popularity of the video affects the hearts of netizens. It turns out that there is more than one "new mom" like her (H. Wang, Trans.). *Xinmin Evening News*. https://sh.qq.com/a/20190422/001359.htm

Xu, Wen. Ed. Chen, Si. (2019, April 23). Mom born in the 1990s "crocheting for handrails" and calling on the society to pay attention to postpartum depression (H. Wang, Trans.). *BJ News*. http://www.bjnews.com.cn/news/2019/04/23/571191.html

Yang, Guobin. (2009). China since Tiananmen: Online activism. *Journal of Democracy, 20*(3), 33–36.

Young mother who suffers from postpartum depression crocheted "sweaters" for the handrails in the entire shopping streets. (2019, May 6) (H. Wang, Trans.). *The People's Daily*. https://baijiahao.baidu.com/s?id=1632751926133738315&wfr=spider&for=pc

#37-year-old overseas female returnee with a PhD, with her 5-month-old daughter,
jumped off the building to death# (April 28, 2020) [Weibo] (H. Wang, Trans.).
https://s.weibo.com/weibo?q=%2337%E5%B2%81%E6%B5%B7%E5%BD%92%
E5%A5%B3%E5%8D%9A%E5%A3%AB%E5%B8%A6%E7%9D%805%E4%B8%
AA%E6%9C%88%E5%A5%B3%E5%84%BF%E8%B7%B3%E6%A5%BC%E8%B-
A%AB%E4%BA%A1%23&Refer=SWeibo_box

7

REROUTING STIGMA

Leading with Law in Mental Health Rhetoric Research

Mark A. Hannah and Susie Salmon

Introduction

In 1981, John W. Hinckley, Jr. attempted to assassinate Ronald Reagan, the President of the United States. At his criminal trial, Hinckley was found not guilty by reason of insanity and confined to a psychiatric hospital instead of prison.[1] Public outrage in the wake of the decision generated a mental health stigma about insanity plea defenses that led to a number of states enacting statutes that narrowed the insanity defense, i.e., shifting the burden of proof or abolishing the defense outright and instead requiring defendants to assert that their mental illnesses deprived them of the requisite *mens rea*, or mental state, for the underlying offenses. Motivated by fears about the threat posed to society by insane defendants walking freely on the streets as well as concerns about defendants "getting off on a technicality" after faking or malingering a mental illness, these statutory changes altered the mental health reality for defendants contemplating an insanity plea. Specifically, they activated and perpetuated the stigma associated with the Hinckley acquittal that rhetorically circulates today (see Hannah & Salmon, 2020) and prefigures defendants with mental illnesses as dangerous, threatening, immoral, and undeserving of the compassion and care that is needed to address their mental health issues. Fast forward nearly 40 years and the mental health stigma associated with the Hinckley acquittal persists today in the law and mental health interface. Some purported advocates for increased funding for mental healthcare and services weaponize and perpetuate this stigma and, instead of focusing public outrage on how systemic failures further marginalize individuals with mental illness, inflame public opinion by tying those failures to sensational violent crimes allegedly committed by individuals with mental illnesses.[2] At the time of this writing, in *Kahler v. Kansas*

DOI: 10.4324/9781003144854-10

(2020), a case with facts that trigger the Hinckley-related stigma, the United States Supreme Court recently affirmed the State of Kansas' right to remove the insanity plea as an affirmative defense. Already vulnerable in the judicial system, those with mental illnesses find themselves further exposed to unjust legal consequences by states' removal of the insanity plea, such as that seen in Kansas.

Though intervening directly in the legal system is difficult for rhetorical scholars due to the law's closed discourse system, this chapter takes seriously the possibility in criminal cases of rhetorical scholars rerouting the stigma associated with insanity plea defenses through cultivating an intermediary role with legal stakeholders—strategic litigators, amicus organizations, and local advocacy offices—in the mental health support network. In particular, we assert that there are opportunities for rhetorical scholars, acting as coproducers of the law (Hannah, 2011), to strategically intervene in impact litigation on the insanity defense and reframe the Hinckley-related stigma that unfavorably casts defendants with mental illnesses as morally unfit and responsible for their actions. Through disrupting the stigmatization process as it appears in legal contexts, our intervention strategy reframes mental health stigma to forestall the onset of such negative perceptions of character that shape legal decision-makers'—judges and jury members—ideas about legal culpability and punishment in the criminal justice system.

In the remainder of this chapter, we set the stage for rhetorical scholars' intervention in the mental health reality of insanity plea criminal cases. We begin with a brief review of stigma-related scholarship in psychology and rhetoric to note the opportunity space for rerouting stigma as a useful mental health intervention strategy. Following the literature review, we describe our rerouting intervention strategy and its underlying rationale. In particular, we discuss the different stages of crafting and participating in impact litigation strategies and specifically note when and how scholars can apply their rhetorical expertise, i.e., rhetorical support work, to reroute stigma away from the echoes of the Hinckley acquittal that prefigures negative perceptions of insanity plea defendants and leaves them in greater jeopardy in criminal proceedings. We then conclude the chapter by briefly discussing hoped-for outcomes of rerouting stigma in mental health rhetoric research.

Situating Stigma in the Law and Mental Health Interface

In this section, we organize stigma literature from psychology and rhetoric around two themes—stigma's roots and rhetorical effects, and stigma in the law and mental health interface—and lay the theoretical groundwork that informs our rhetorical intervention for rerouting stigma in mental health rhetoric research.

Stigma's Roots and Rhetorical Effects

As a psychological concept, stigma has received much scholarly attention since Erving Goffman (1963) first coined the phrase "spoiled identity" to represent how the public perceived and understood those with mental illnesses (Corrigan et al., 2014; Johnson, 2010). For Goffman, the core feature of stigmatization was how it socially discredited those individuals and led them to being perceived as dangerous and unpredictable, responsible for their illness, and incompetent to handle daily tasks like working or living independently (Corrigan, 2004; Corrigan et al., 2014; Johnson, 2010; Krendl & Freeman, 2019). Through such "labelling" (Angermeyer & Matschinger, 2003; Corrigan, 2004), these individuals experienced discrimination in various ways, such as: poor access to mental healthcare, exclusion from education and employment opportunities, victimization, and increased risks of contact with the criminal justice system (Gronholm et al., 2017). Concerned about such harms, mental health researchers and practitioners sought to remove and/or mitigate mental health stigma through protest, education, and contact intervention strategies (Corrigan & Penn, 1999; Corrigan, 2004; Thornicroft et al., 2016); however, due to the persistence of stigma, these interventions had limited effects (Gronholm et al., 2017); education generally being the most successful in only fostering short-term mitigation of stigmatizing attitudes (Thornicroft et al., 2016). Together, the body of psychological and mental health research demonstrates that mental health stigma is a pervasive, ongoing problem unlikely to be eliminated (Corrigan & Penn, 1999; Molloy, 2015; Molloy, Holladay, & Melonçon, 2020). Despite this resilience, though, calls for antistigma programs persist in the mental health landscape with particular emphasis on countering stereotypes, most notably in regards to weakness and craziness labels, and lessening judgment and rejection of people with mental health problems (Clement et al., 2015).[3]

Drawing from this body of psychological and mental health research, rhetoricians focus their work not only on understanding stigma's resiliency and how it denies opportunities to those with mental illnesses but also on understanding how stigma influences their rhetorical, communicative capacity. As a phenomenon, stigma is both rhetorically constituted and rhetorically disabling (Johnson, 2010; Prendergast, 2001). More specifically, stigma is created, shaped, and spread by communication; furthermore, communication can be used to stigmatize, devalue, and ostracize individuals with mental illnesses and ultimately deny them their rhetorical agency or rhetoricity (Lewiecki-Wilson, 2003; Smith, Zhu, & Quesnell, 2016). The denial of rhetoricity is sustained when stigma undermines and discredits a mentally disabled person's ethos or character, especially in instances when a mentally disabled person's condition is disclosed (Johnson, 2010; Prendergast, 2001; Uthappa, 2017).

Despite the rhetorical harm caused by mental health stigma, there are opportunities for mentally disabled individuals to recuperate and possibly restore their rhetoricity and attendant ethos (Johnson, 2010; Molloy, 2015). For example, Cynthia Lewiecki-Wilson (2003) argued that rhetoricity could be restored if the concept were expanded to include acts of mediated rhetoricity that emerge when a mentally disabled individual's support network (i.e., parents, advocates, and caregivers) uses language for the benefit of that person. Ultimately, these collaborative communicative acts enable mentally disabled individuals to recover their voice through speaking "with/out language" (Lewiecki-Wilson, 2003, p. 27). Lastly, while not explicitly about mental health stigma, Dan Brouwer's (1998) analysis of stigma associated with HIV/AIDS tattoos makes a compelling case for the possibility of cultivating what Cathryn Molloy (2015) later coined as "recuperative ethos." Specifically, he noted that through being seen, a self-stigmatizer has the potential to accrue greater social, political, and cultural legitimacy; on the other hand, he also noted that in voluntarily making oneself visible, a person also summons surveillance and the law and thus creates conditions for undermining their ethos yet again. Brouwer's recognition of law in this instance is relevant to mental health rhetoric research in that it alludes to law's always already responsive nature. That is, rhetorical action, even if not explicitly intended by a rhetor, will call forth law's potentially constraining, determinative nature that will name and fix a rhetor's behaviors in a legal category (Andrus, 2015; Hannah et al., 2021; McKinnon, 2016) that will be used to evaluate and draw legal conclusions about such action. Despite this potential limitation, though, Brouwer (1998) and Lewiecki-Wilson's (2003) work reveals opportunities for those with mental illnesses to engage in affirmative, collaborative rhetorical action that reframes their rhetorical ability as constitutive rather than merely disabled.

Stigma, Law, and Mental Health

Though not extensive, psychological and rhetorical research do address the influence of stigma in the law and mental health interface. Historically, the assumed connection between mental illness and immorality led to the jailing of those with mental illnesses. In some instances, those individuals were put to death (Corrigan, 2002; Overton & Medina, 2008). Over time, stigma became more entrenched in society's social structures and influenced the ways law, social services, and the justice system were structured as well as how mental health resources were allocated (Corrigan & Watson, 2002). For example, as mental illness was criminalized, the police, rather than mental health professionals, became the primary responders to mental health crises (Corrigan, 2004), a decision that has significantly heightened the further deinstitutionalization of mental health services (Gronholm et al., 2017). Operating outside institutional settings, stigma shaped how citizens call forth and/or respond to perceived criminal behavior. For instance, studies have documented how citizens discriminate against individuals with mental illnesses by being more likely to falsely press charges against them for violent crimes (Corrigan & Penn, 1999). Further compounding the influence of mental health stigma in legal contexts are popular media representations of mental illness that forward through their language choices the idea that those with mental illnesses are violent and prone to criminality. Examples of this terminology include terms and phrases like homicidal maniacs, psychopath, nutter, and wacko (Corrigan & Penn, 1999; Harper, 2005; Sieff, 2003). Together, these institutional factors, citizen behaviors, and popular media representations fundamentally shape the mental health reality in which defendants with mental illnesses contemplate an insanity plea, and it is from this background that our intervention strategy emerges.

Rerouting through Strategic Litigation

One way rhetorical scholars could engage with law as coproducers to reroute mental health stigma would be to participate in various stages of impact litigation on the insanity defense. Although in some instances the attorney's ethically mandated objective of asserting legal and factual arguments that best protect and advance the client's interests may not align perfectly with rhetoricians' goal of rerouting stigma, by contributing rhetorical expertise and engaging in a nonprescriptive dialogue with the attorneys early and repeatedly in a litigation process, rhetorical scholars can impact the extent to which the litigation and any resulting legal decisions reinforce or reroute stigma. In this section, we discuss the following interventions and their attendant rhetorical support work within impact litigation:

- Identifying the Issue
- Identifying the Client and Case
- The Litigation Itself—shaping written communication; shaping oral communication; and framing the theme and theory of the case

Before identifying the intervention opportunities, though, it helps to have an overall understanding of what impact litigation is, how it works, and the various stages at which rhetorical intervention may be possible and fruitful.

In general, attorneys engage in litigation to vindicate the rights of individual clients. But in impact litigation—sometimes called strategic litigation or cause lawyering—attorneys identify and pursue legal cases with an eye to achieving goals that go beyond the issues facing an individual client and seek to affect broader, sustained, and sometimes systemic change (Klarman, 2009). Often, impact litigation aims to advance human rights by bringing about significant changes in law, policy, public perception, or all three. Probably the most famous strategic litigation campaign—and the one on which much subsequent impact litigation has been modeled—is the one masterminded by Thurgood Marshall and conducted by lawyers with the NAACP Legal Defense and Education Fund that culminated in the ruling in *Brown v. Board of Education* (1954), overturning the "separate but equal" doctrine.

High-profile impact litigation not only affects the law, but it can also affect public opinion through media coverage. Regardless of the outcome of the litigation, media coverage of that litigation can draw attention to injustices, spark outrage, motivate action, and provoke or influence a national or international dialogue about an issue. In the insanity defense context, this is especially useful as the media is the primary means through which the public learns about mental health (Sieff, 2003). Rhetorical scholars' support in both crafting media messaging and identifying kairotic openings to place such messaging within the impact litigation process can have significant influence in rerouting the persistent Hinckley-related stigma. For example, developing and deploying language attuned to the barriers—social, economic, education, legal—that constrain the mental health reality for those with mental illnesses can draw attention away from stigmatizing labels like crazy or wacko. In doing so, rhetorical scholars enable reframing efforts that embed within the public imaginary ideas about individuals with mental illnesses as actively participating in the public sphere rather than threatening it with their presence. Admittedly, like earlier education intervention strategies, educating through media may have limited success, but the initial hoped-for mitigation will generate the kind of rhetorical momentum necessary to move the impact litigation process forward.

Impact litigation may take the form of a class action, or it may involve a single plaintiff. In either instance, although only the parties to the litigation are directly bound by the court's ruling, the holding from the case at the appellate or Supreme Court level becomes law that binds courts in future cases. Impact litigation organizations often engage in litigation as third parties by filing *amicus curiae*—"friend of the court"—briefs in cases that involve issues related to the organization's overall mission. Most commonly used in matters before the United States Supreme Court, amicus briefs are filed by entities that have an interest in the issues relevant to a litigation but are not parties to that litigation. Amicus briefs often serve an educational role. Unlike parties to the litigation, authors of amicus briefs have wide latitude to present to the Court facts—such as medical or sociological research—that were not introduced in the trial court but that might inform the Court's understanding of the issues, put the case in a context, and illuminate the broader impacts of a ruling. One famous example of an amicus brief that sought to educate the Court regarding the broader context of the case was what came to be known as the "Brandeis Brief," filed by then-attorney Louis Brandeis in a case arguing for a limited workday for women. The Brandeis Brief provided the Court with sociological studies and medical and economic data not introduced by the parties in the underlying litigation.

A number of organizations such as Mental Health Advocacy Services and the Judge David L. Bazelon Center for Mental Health Law do impact litigation in the mental health arena. Rhetorical scholars could collaborate with these organizations and apply their expertise in evaluating a network of rhetorical situations (Hannah & Salmon, 2020), reframing issues, developing multimodal arguments, and applying medical information in a Brandeis-style amicus brief. This kind of support work would aim to bring in contextual information as well as value systems that the law tries to exclude (Campbell, 1983; Hannah & Salmon, 2020; Rand, 2015). Overall, the primary aim of this work is recuperating the defendants' ethos via "mediated rhetoricity" and helping them recover their voice that effectively was lost the moment the insanity plea was made and the Hinckley-related stigma began to speak for them. Logistically, rhetorical scholars might engage in this process as expert consultants on a litigation team, board members, or as volunteers with advocacy organizations.

For the purposes of the advice in this chapter, it helps to think of impact litigation as having three phases that present intervention opportunities for rhetorical scholars: identifying the cause or issue, identifying the client and case, and the actual litigation itself.

Identifying the Issue

First, the organization must identify a specific issue to pursue. Of course, impact litigation organizations generally operate in alignment with broad animating principles, for example, Lambda Legal's mission of "achieving full recognition of the civil rights of lesbians, gay men, bisexuals, transgender people, and everyone living with HIV" (n.d.), or the NAACP Legal Defense Fund's (LDF) (2020) mission of "seeking structural changes to expand democracy, eliminate disparities, and achieve racial justice in a society that fulfills the promise of all Americans." However, when an issue is narrower and represents an incremental, strategic step toward advancing the underlying mission, additionally, each issue may include multiple subissues. For example, the NAACP LDF has identified "barriers to voting" as an issue. Subissues of voting barriers include time frames for voter registration, mandatory identification, state voter-roll-purge programs, the use of provisional ballots, and voter intimidation and suppression tactics. The NAACP LDF might bring litigation regarding aspects of any of those subissues with the ultimate goal of incrementally advancing the larger issue and thus its overall mission. The opportunity for rhetorical scholars to collaborate in the support network when identifying an issue stems from their partitioning expertise, specifically the ability to break down a concept into its constitutive parts and note their relationality (Johnson-Sheehan, 2017). For example, regarding mental health treatment, the rhetorical scholar could partition and map (Sullivan & Porter, 1997) the medical, political, social, economic, cultural, and legal dimensions and put them in conversation to demonstrate how they influence and/or constitute each other. Part of partitioning expertise is rhetorical scholars' ability to strategically name each dimension to signal its primary function. The concern with naming is akin to how lawyers translate and name events and facts into legal categories. Rhetorical scholars' contribution in naming here would not be to replace the legal category that makes the particular dimension legally intelligible (Andrus, 2015; Hannah et al., 2021, McKinnon, 2016). Rather, the contribution would be in working to contextualize the legal category when it later will be discussed in the brief. Again, this kind of support work would bring in the contextual elements and value systems that law works to exclude.

In the case of an impact litigation organization seeking to revive a true insanity defense in a way that comports with the realities of those living with mental illness while also rerouting the stigma associated with the defense, the organization might identify incremental subissues to pursue through targeted cases. At this stage, rhetorical scholars might consult with those identifying subissues to steer them towards naming issues that provide the opportunity to reframe the definition of insanity for the purposes of the defense, crafting a legal standard that not only honors the latest mental health research but also employs phrasing that reroutes rather than reinforces stigma. Even though any advocacy regarding changes to the legal standard must also evaluate both the research on juror decision-making in cases where the insanity defense is raised and recommendations by experts in the mental health community, including the American Psychiatric Association and organizations like Mental Health America, rhetoric scholars could, for example, suggest language that focuses less on public safety or fears of recidivism and steers decision-makers toward competent, comprehensive expert testimony regarding the defendant's mental state at the time of the offense might better accomplish both goals.

Identifying the Client and Case

Once they identify an issue, organizations engaged in impact litigation choose cases and clients carefully in hopes of obtaining a more favorable outcome. A sympathetic client to whom the court can relate may be able to exploit the court's biases and predispositions to obtain a ruling in the client's favor, thereby creating legal precedent that will affect future cases—even those with less sympathetic parties—favorably. For example, in *Weinberger v. Wiesenfeld* (1975), then-law professor Ruth Bader Ginsburg represented a male plaintiff in attacking gender-based distinctions under the Social Security Act, obtaining an opinion that ultimately helped advance the cause of greater gender equality. Selecting a case with a male plaintiff—who sat next to Ginsburg during oral argument—arguably made the gender discrimination issue more relatable to the eight men on the Supreme Court who participated in the unanimous opinion.

The adage that "bad facts make bad law" often proves true; as a result, impact litigators are careful to choose a case where the facts tend to make the decision-maker feel that the outcome the impact litigators seek will serve the ends of justice and fairness. The *Kahler v. Kansas* (2020) case, discussed in the Introduction, for example, does not provide such facts: on Thanksgiving weekend, a few months after his wife sought divorce and moved from their house with their three children, the defendant drove to his wife's grandmother's house, shot and killed his wife, then hunted down the other women in the house, including his two daughters and his wife's grandmother, and shot and killed them as well. The facts of that case triggered both aspects of the insanity stigma: the defendant's acts invoke images of a murderous madman run amok in the sacred safety of a family home, and his targeting of his estranged wife and the other female members of the family might lead some to conclude that his acts were compelled not by mental illness, but by revenge, a hatred of women, or a laundry list of other motives that align him with killers like Elliot Rodger,[4] who loom large in the public imagination and dialogue about mental illness and violence.

The opportunity for rhetorical scholars in identifying a client and case stems from their expertise in audience analysis and rhetorical situation analysis. Regarding the former, scholars could collaborate with the impact litigation team to think through the different levels of audience—primary, secondary, tertiary—and identify the distinct ways in which audiences might respond to the facts and circumstances of a particular insanity defendant's case. As part of this analysis, rhetorical scholars would help the team think through the information needs of each audience type and select evidence attuned to their respective needs. In insanity cases, where medical information is of many types—psychological, neurological, behavioral, physical, historical—and varying levels of complexity, this skill is especially relevant when demonstrating through written argument that a defendant is treatable and better served by confinement to a mental health facility rather than prison. Complementing audience analysis, rhetorical scholars' expertise in assessing rhetorical situations will broaden the impact litigation team's ability to understand what factors are impacting a defendant's case. In particular, rhetorical scholars can articulate how the Hinckley-related stigma rhetorically circulates to the case at hand and potentially influences perceptions of the defendant. Armed with this knowledge, the litigation team can reroute those aspects of the stigma that foster negative perceptions by demonstrating how the defendant is unlike Hinckley and the prior string of defendants shaped by the Hinckley stigma.

For impact litigators in the criminal defense arena, most often the case and defendant selection process would occur when determining in which cases to assist on appeal, whether through amicus briefing or through handling the appeal itself. Ideally, in an insanity defense case, the impact litigators would choose a defendant and a factual scenario that do not trigger the decision-maker's preconceived notions about what a dangerously insane person looks or acts like or suggest malingering or dishonesty. A rhetorical scholar could help at this stage by participating on a case selection board, sensitizing the attorneys making these decisions to the stigma, and advising on the types of defendants and fact scenarios that might reinforce or reroute that stigma.

The Litigation Itself

The actual litigation presents at least three types of intervention opportunities: opportunities to shape written communication, opportunities to shape oral communication, and opportunities to frame the theme and theory of the case that influence both the written and the oral communication. These opportunities present whether rhetorical scholars collaborate with an impact litigation organization or simply consult with counsel on particular cases involving the insanity defense.

Good litigators develop a theory of the case for every litigation. The theory of the case is a narrative that accounts for the undisputed facts and governing law in a way that comports with common sense and will appeal to the judge or jury, making the client sympathetic. The theory of the case also frames the outcome the attorney seeks as the one most consistent with fairness and justice. Ideally, the theory is engaging and simple enough to summarize in a single paragraph and be understood by an individual of ordinary intelligence. The theme is shorter—perhaps a sentence, a phrase, or even just a word or two— and captures the theory clearly and memorably. Good litigators formulate both the theory of the case and theme early in the litigation, and both inform everything that follows, from witness examination to the vocabulary the attorneys use in briefing and oral argument. In the *Brown* (1954) case, for example, the simple but powerful theme of "separate is inherently unequal" both effectively countered the prevailing law—that separate but equal facilities were lawful— and so resonated with all audiences that Chief Justice Warren echoed it in his opinion and it became the mantra of desegregationists for years to come.

Because the theory of the case and theme will affect all written and oral communication in the litigation, an intervention by rhetorical scholars at this stage can have significant impact. Within the constraints of the legal standards and relevant facts, rhetorical scholars can support invention work for narratives that comport with those standards and facts while also rerouting stigma about individuals who assert the insanity defense. Through mediated rhetoricity, this invention work again focuses on articulating defendants' efforts to combat stigma by attempting to work through the barriers in daily life that deny them rights and opportunities available to the general population. The rhetorical scholar might have even more impact in invention work by developing themes that advance the legally necessary narrative of lack of culpability, i.e., that the defendant acted reasonably in light of the facts and circumstances of the case, while still recuperating the defendant's ethos and restoring the defendant's voice and attendant ability to assert nondangerousness and essential morality.

Whether at the trial or appellate stage, the attorneys will write briefs that frame legal and factual issues for court. Although to some extent what the attorneys write is constrained by the legal theories available, any legally significant language they need to use, and the facts at issue, attorneys do have some latitude in how they frame the facts and legal issues and the vocabulary they use in doing so. Particularly at the appellate level, the attorney also exercises discretion regarding which legal theories to pursue, which legal arguments to make, and how much "airtime" to give particular arguments. A rhetorical scholar could participate in the briefing in a number of ways. Before the attorney or attorneys begin writing the brief, the rhetorical scholar could again participate in the impact litigation team's invention work and provide advice and general guidelines—dos and don'ts, as it were—on vocabulary and framing issues. An attorney is bound by the ethical rules to state all legally relevant facts, and in general legal knowledge is required to identify what those are, but rhetorical scholars could advise on the language to use in describing the larger rhetorical context, e.g., the client generally, the client's mental illness, and the client's acts. In this description, as in previous intervention work, rhetorical scholars would advise on how to bring in contextual factors and related values that further explicate the defendant's particularized situation as distinct from the circulating, generalized Hinckley facts that in effect coalesce all insanity defendants into an undifferentiated collection of cases. Lastly, when the attorney must respond to the opponent's brief, rhetorical scholars can apply their expertise in discourse analysis (Gee, 2014) and identify problematic language or framing in that brief and provide suggestions for countering those issues in the response brief.

Finally, attorneys engage in oral communication that provides opportunities for rhetorical scholars to intervene in the impact litigation process. Before virtually any appellate oral argument—and certainly before any argument in front of the United States Supreme Court—the attorney who will deliver the argument participates in a number of "moots" to rehearse and fine-tune the argument. Often, other attorneys in the organization—whether they were involved in the case itself or not—will serve as mock appellate judges, grilling the advocate with questions designed to anticipate challenges the real tribunal might pose. During or after each moot, those who acted as mock judges and others who may simply have observed the argument provide constructive feedback to the advocate. Sometimes this feedback relies on legal knowledge; often, however, it falls more in the vein of workshopping how answers are phrased or arguments are framed to make them more persuasive to the court. The moot presents some obvious ways for rhetorical scholars to collaborate with the litigation team. They could participate in one or more moots leading up to the oral argument, helping to guide how the attorney frames and phrases the facts or issues or responses to anticipated questions for the court or arguments advanced by opposing counsel in a way that reroutes stigma.

Taken together, these three phases of an impact litigation strategy offer rhetorical scholars a variety of intervention points for addressing stigma in insanity defense contexts. Though presented here as distinct phases, it is important to understand them as in conversation and operating relationally to spur rerouting activities. Developing a concerted and coordinated effort with the litigation team will require some professional networking[5] and negotiation of disciplinary power and case-making about rhetorical expertise (Hannah & Arreguin, 2017; Henning & Bemer, 2016), but the potential for impact requires rhetorical scholars' tenacious involvement in asserting their power and legitimacy (Kynell-Hunt & Savage, 2003; St. Amant & Melonçon, 2016) in promoting just ends in mental health rhetoric research.

Deactivating Mental Health

As noted extensively in the literature, stigma is difficult and perhaps even impossible to mitigate. As a rhetorical practice, rerouting via partnering with strategic litigation teams is a needed intervention strategy for addressing stigma in insanity plea contexts. Our hope with this intervention strategy is that it produces long-lasting impacts beyond the slight success seen in prior protest, education, and contact change strategies. Achieving such impact, though, will require a deactivation of the Hinckley acquittal's pernicious effects in order to create space for those with mental illnesses to operate in, recuperate their ethos, and ultimately regain their rhetoricity. Such change undoubtedly will take time, but in the meantime, rhetorical scholars can intervene in strategic litigation teams and begin creating and fostering conditions for the kinds of rerouting work that is needed for the required deactivation to occur. Once achieved, insanity plea defendants and their legal teams can lead with both law and rhetorical expertise in crafting a persuasive legal defense.

Notes

1 "Insanity is the legal concept of a severe mental illness or condition causing a lack of competence or guilt. Generally, not guilty by reason of insanity means having committed but not being responsible for the crime charged due to severe mental illness causing a lack of guilt. The plea of not guilty by reason of insanity is the plea of an accused that the accused committed but is not responsible for the crime charged due to severe mental illness causing a lack of guilt" (Nolfi, 2008).
2 See, e.g., E. Fuller Torrey (2008).
3 Though persistent, empirical data (Pescosolido & Martin, 2015) suggests that some anti-stigma campaigns, like education, likely represent a waste of scarce and valuable resources, and thus implies a need to innovate beyond traditional approaches through interventions like rerouting discussed in this chapter.

4 On May 23, 2014, near the University of California, Santa Barbara campus, Elliot Rodger killed six people by gunshot and stabbing, injured 14 others, and then later killed himself. Roger described his motivation as both his desire to punish women for rejecting him and his envy of sexually active men.

5 When thinking about how to expand their professional networks to connect with legal communities, rhetorical scholars might consider working from a micro to macro perspective. That is, rhetorical scholars can begin locally at their home institutions and reach out to individuals in departments such as psychology, criminal justice, business, and political science that have coursework and/or projects that directly engage with law. Through those contacts, rhetorical scholars can begin developing a sense of the lay of the land about the kinds of issues that potentially animate mental health law issues. At the same time, rhetorical scholars can ask for guidance about how to broaden their emerging legal-rhetoric professional network beyond their home institutions and begin connecting with legal stakeholders and decision-makers working at the state and local levels. Through these extra-institutional contacts, rhetorical scholars can initiate conversations and begin exploring how mental health law issues show up in and shape the conditions of everyday life. In these conversations, rhetorical scholars can investigate how these contacts perform their own networking with mental health stakeholders, specifically as to how they foster relationships with local, national, and international collaborators that support their work. It is at this point when rhetorical scholars can begin modeling not only how to cultivate the relationships that are required to perform the kinds of interventions discussed in this chapter but also how to make the case for the very rhetorical support work that embodies successful interventions in mental health contexts regarding the insanity defense.

References

Andrus, Jennifer. (2015). *Entextualizing domestic violence: Language ideology and violence against women in the Anglo-American hearsay principle.* Oxford University Press.

Angermeyer, Matthias C., & Matschinger, Herbert. (2003). The stigma of mental illness: Effects of labelling on public attitudes towards people with mental disorder. *Acta Psychiatrica Scandinavica, 108*(4), 304–309.

Brouwer, Dan. (1998). The precarious visibility politics of self-stigmatization: The case of HIV/AIDS tattoos. *Text and Performance Quarterly, 18*(2), 114–136.

Brown v. Board of Education of Topeka, 347 U.S. 483. (1954). https://www.oyez.org/cases/1940-1955/347us483

Campbell, J. Louis. (1983). The spirit of dissent. *Judicature, 66*(7), 304–312.

Clement, Sarah, Schauman, Oliver, Graham, Tanya, Maggioni, F., Evans-Lacko, Sara, Bezborodovs, Nikita, Morgan, Craig, Rüsch, Nicolas, Brown, June S. L., & Thornicroft, Graham. (2015). What is the impact of mental health-related stigma on help-seeking? A systematic review of quantitative and qualitative studies. *Psychological Medicine, 45*(1), 11–27.

Corrigan, Patrick W. (2002). Empowerment and serious mental illness: Treatment partnerships and community opportunities. *Psychiatric Quarterly, 73*(3), 217–228. doi:10.1023/a:1016040805432

Corrigan, Patrick W. (2004). How stigma interferes with mental health care. *American Psychologist, 59*(7), 614.

Corrigan, Patrick W., Druss, Benjamin G., & Perlick, Deborah A. (2014). The impact of mental illness stigma on seeking and participating in mental health care. *Psychological Science in the Public Interest, 15*(2), 37–70. doi:10.1177/1529100614531398

Corrigan, Patrick W., & Penn, David L. (1999). Lessons from social psychology on discrediting psychiatric stigma. *Stigma and Health, 1*(S), 2. doi:10.1037//0003066x.54.9.765

Corrigan, Patrick W., & Watson, Amy C. (2002). Understanding the impact of stigma on people with mental illness. *World Psychiatry, 1*(1), 16.

Gee, James P. (2014). *An introduction to discourse analysis: Theory and method.* Routledge.

Goffman, Erving. (1963). *Stigma: Notes on the management of spoiled identity.* Simon and Shuster.

Gronholm, Petra C., Henderson, Claire, Deb, Tanya, & Thornicroft, Graham. (2017). Interventions to reduce discrimination and stigma: The state of the art. *Social Psychiatry and Psychiatric Epidemiology, 52*(3), 249–258.

Hannah, Mark A. (2011). Legal literacy: Coproducing the law in technical communication. *Technical Communication Quarterly, 20*(1), 5–24.

Hannah, Mark A., & Arreguin, Alex. (2017). Cultivating conditions for access: A case for "case-making" in graduate student preparation for interdisciplinary research. *Journal of Technical Writing and Communication, 47*(2), 172–193.

Hannah, Mark A., Moore, Kristen. R., Alonge, Kehinde, & Lowman, Nicole. (2021). Legal resource mapping as a methodology for social justice research and engagement. In Rebecca Walton, & Godwin Y. Agboka (Eds.), *Equipping technical communicators for social justice work: Theories, methods, and topics* (pp. 74–96). Utah State University Press.

Hannah, Mark A., & Salmon, Susie. (2020). Against the grain: The secret role of dissents in integrating rhetoric across the curriculum. *Nevada Law Journal, 20*(3), 935–966.

Harper, Stephen. (2005). Media, madness and misrepresentation: Critical reflections on anti-stigma discourse. *European Journal of Communication, 20*(4), 460–483.

Henning, Teresa, & Bemer, Amanda. (2016). Reconsidering power and legitimacy in technical communication: A case for enlarging the definition of technical communicator. *Journal of Technical Writing and Communication, 46*(3), 311–341.

Johnson, Jenell. (2010). The skeleton on the couch: The Eagleton affair, rhetorical disability, and the stigma of mental illness. *Rhetoric Society Quarterly, 40*(5), 459–478.

Johnson-Sheehan, Richard. (2017). *Technical communication today.* 6th ed. Pearson/Longman.

Kahler v. Kansas, 589 U.S. ___ (2020). https://www.oyez.org/cases/2019/18-6135

Klarman, Michael J. (2009). Social reform litigation and its challenges: An essay in honor of Justice Ruth Bader Ginsburg. *Harvard Journal of Law & Gender, 32*, 251.

Krendl, Anne C., & Freeman, Jonathan B. (2019). Are mental illnesses stigmatized for the same reasons? Identifying the stigma-related beliefs underlying common mental illnesses. *Journal of Mental Health, 28*(3), 267–275.

Kynell-Hunt, Teresa, & Savage, Gerald J. (2003). *Power and legitimacy in technical communication: The historical and contemporary struggle for professional status* (Vol. 1). Baywood Publishing Company.

Lambda Legal. (n.d.). *About us.* https://www.lambdalegal.org/about-us

Lewiecki-Wilson, Cynthia. (2003). Rethinking rhetoric through mental disabilities. *Rhetoric Review, 22*(2), 156–167.

McKinnon, Sara L. (2016). *Gendered asylum: Race and violence in US law and politics.* University of Illinois Press.

Molloy, Cathryn. (2015). Recuperative ethos and agile epistemologies: Toward a vernacular engagement with mental illness ontologies. *Rhetoric Society Quarterly, 45*(2), 138–163.

Molloy, Cathryn, Holladay, Drew, & Melonçon, Lisa. (2020). The place of mental health rhetoric research (MHRR) in rhetoric of health and medicine and beyond. *Rhetoric of Health & Medicine, 3*(2), iii–x.

NAACP Legal Defense and Educational Fund, Inc. (2020). *About us.* https://www.naacpldf.org/about-us/

Nolfi, Edward. (2008). *Legal terminology explained.* McGraw-Hill Higher Education.

Overton, Stacy L., & Medina, Sondra L. (2008). The stigma of mental illness. *Journal of Counseling & Development, 86*(2), 143–151.

Pescosolido, Bernice A., & Martin, Jack K. (2015). The stigma complex. *Annual Review of Sociology, 41*, 87–116.

Prendergast, Catherine. J. (2001). On the rhetorics of mental disability. In James C. Wilson, & Cynthia Lewiecki-Wilson (Eds.), *Embodied rhetorics: Disability in language and culture* (pp. 45–60). Southern Illinois University Press.

Rand, Erin J. (2015). Fear the frill: Ruth Bader Ginsburg and the uncertain futurity of feminist judicial dissent. *Quarterly Journal of Speech, 101*(1), 72–84.

Sieff, Elaine. (2003). Media frames of mental illnesses: The potential impact of negative frames. *Journal of Mental Health, 12*(3), 259–269.

Smith, Rachel A., Zhu, Xun, & Quesnell, Madisen. (2016). Stigma and health/risk communication. *Oxford Research Encyclopedia of Communication.*

St. Amant, Kirk, & Melonçon, Lisa. (2016). Addressing the incommensurable: A research-based perspective for considering issues of power and legitimacy in the field. *Journal of Technical Writing and Communication, 46*(3), 267–283.

Sullivan, Patricia, & Porter, James E. (1997). *Opening spaces: Writing technologies and critical research practices.* Greenwood Publishing Group.

Thornicroft, Graham, Mehta, Nisha, Clement, Sarah, Evans-Lacko, Sara, Doherty, Mary, Rose, Diana, Koschorke, Mirja, Shidhaye, Rahul, O'Reilly, Claire, & Henderson, Claire. (2016). Evidence for effective interventions to reduce mental health-related stigma and discrimination. *The Lancet, 387*(10023), 1123–1132.

Torrey, E. Fuller (2008). *The insanity offense: How America's failure to treat the seriously mentally ill endangers its citizens.* W.W. Norton & Company, Inc.

Uthappa, N. Renuka. (2017). Moving closer: Speakers with mental disabilities, deep disclosure, and agency through vulnerability. *Rhetoric Review, 36*(2), 164–175.

Weinberger v. Wiesenfeld, 420 U.S. 636. (1975). https://www.oyez.org/cases/1974/73-1892.

8

DESTIGMATIZING BLACK MENTAL HEALTH

A Black Gay Woman's Experience

Tianna Cobb

Introduction: My Experiences, My Approach

> I was ten. On the left side, I sat in the last pew, closest to the middle aisle. I listened—he preached, "… and if you're gay or man on man or woman on woman, you are not welcomed here. The Lord does not love you." He said more, but I couldn't hear anything else—just silence. My head dropped, and my eyebrows scrunched together as I tried to hold it all back. But then…tears slowly traveled down my little cheeks.

"Why are you here?" That is the question that popped into my mind when I first walked through my therapist's doors. The query yielded some of the most complex emotions I had felt. I could pinpoint pivotal moments that have taken a toll on my mental health, but I also knew there was more. There were more experiences that I have blocked from my memory, more behaviors I excused, and healthier actions I continuously put off. I knew my biggest battle was internal, but I was unsure if I was ready to unpack everything I believed I was protecting myself from. However, that in itself was self-deception. Honestly, when is one ever truly prepared for that kind of honesty and self-reflection?

I had many moments of revelation that led me to seeing my therapist. Now reflecting, I can recognize the compilation of experiences that shaped my thoughts, perceptions, and behaviors. As they say, hindsight is 20/20. Then, I was unaware of how those experiences affected me. I thought keeping everything inside was the best way to protect myself. Honestly, I believed that was the best way to deal with everything, until I could not hold it in anymore. Then I knew something needed to change. Instead of processing my trauma,

DOI: 10.4324/9781003144854-11

I was masking it. It was starting to spill over into other aspects of my life. I could see that trauma in my work, my relationships with other people, and most importantly, my relationship with myself. If I did not change something soon, I was going to self-destruct. My cup was overflowing. Honestly, it had been overflowing for some time. I reached my emotional limit over and over again. Why did it take so long for me to shift my perception and start my healing journey?

The way I coped with trauma was normal to me. That was how my family dealt with their problems. I learned that we were being strong. I learned it was enough to just make it through the day and to the next. I learned I needed to protect everyone else by dealing with my own problems. I learned I needed to shift my actions to make situations more ideal for other people. I learned to remain quiet about family issues. I learned I could trust no one. I learned I had to work twice as hard as my counterparts. I learned I had to hide parts of myself to make others comfortable. I learned I had to dress a certain way to get noticed. I learned I had to speak a certain way. I learned I had to wear my hair a certain way. I learned I had to keep my calm at all times. I learned I could not trust doctors. I learned I could not trust religious leaders. I learned I could not trust the White man—he was always out to get us. I learned all of this from a young age. As I grew older, I learned even more about the social, political, and economic consequences of my race, gender, and sexual orientation. I implemented these behaviors in my life without understanding why, the costs, or that I could change it.

Before therapy, I did not possess the tools needed to comb through my past experiences and connect them to my current. I did not realize how impactful my past was on my present. We all hear the saying that "hurt people hurt people." Traumatized people inflict trauma onto others, often subconsciously. People often treat others how they are treated. People often parent how they were parented. People often approach relationships based on those they witnessed. The correlations go on and on. This is not to say that people are intentional in causing emotional harm to others or themselves. Regardless of whether people can decipher a behavior as right or wrong, if they have no recollection of a healthier alternative, they choose the most viable option based on experience. Once alternatives arise, people are presented with options to choose from regarding future paths. As a teacher and researcher, I have realized the power that resides within each of us to share alternative paths with others through a connection of shared experiences. That is what this chapter is about. Before getting into the particulars of the argument, though, I want to step back and offer some ruminations on how I approached this work, how it relates to larger antiracist projects, and how I grappled with asserting my own voice and experiences in an academic venue.

In preparing for this chapter, I went through many obstacles trying to organize my thoughts and intertwine my experiences with existing literature. In academia, people tell you to read more when you are having difficulty writing. It is assumed that reading more leads to a clearer perspective (Curthoys & McGrath, 2011; Lee, 2005). So, I read more. Every time I hit a roadblock in my writing, I read. The problem was despite my continual reading, I was still unable to write with clear direction. That was when I realized—it was not the amount I was reading, but what I was reading. Initially, I was reading academic articles and books on mental health inequities, mental health rhetoric, mental health and the Black community, and other mostly academic sources. I was used to the academic style of writing. So, I was drawn to those pieces first, but I was not connecting to these texts as a writer for this particular chapter. It was not until I was referred to sources such as Tressie McMillian Cottom's (2018) *Thick: and Other Essays* and Rasheedah Phillips, Iresha Picot, and Vanessa Hazzard's (2015) *The Color of Hope: People of Color Mental Health Narratives*, that I was able to hit my creative stride and organize my thoughts and experiences. Those works underscore and guide the writing and my approach to "argument" in this piece.

As a primarily qualitative researcher, I add to existing literature and theoretical perspectives by sharing others' stories and experiences through data. However, as a researcher, I still have some level of distance between myself and the data. As a critical scholar, I also know that not all experiences are accurately represented, or represented at all, within research. Further, when some marginalized experiences are shared, power dynamics regarding the dissemination of certain studies and scholars minimize such research exposure. As a result, the research may not receive recognition itself, let alone get the opportunity to build upon research representative of those communities. Therefore, people of color, and more specifically the Black community, have too few opportunities to come across studies to which they connect on a personal level.

I have been trained mostly in qualitative scholarship, more specifically interpretive. This preparation has led me to be a bit strict regarding my work's structure and rigor. While interpretive scholars acknowledge that social reality is intersubjective and exists amongst the researcher themselves, there are still measures taken to ensure collection and analysis methods are valid and reliable. I have learned, however, that such distance is impossible in sharing my story and may not necessarily be most effective. My standpoint aligns with the epistemological perspective that many social realities exist based on our experiences. While my formal training in interpretive studies has helped me to develop as a scholar, I've also relied on the critical work I've come across from my peers and via my own research. My stance, thus, aligns with the critical perspective that some social realities are constrained due to hegemonic marginalization. While most scholars try to remain objective and separate from the concept of "power," the two are historically entangled (Delgado & Stefancic, 2017). Indeed, one reality does not exist without the other. Therefore, accounts of social realities are merely fragments of little "t" truths when examined separately from power.

As a Black woman who is gay, focusing on objectivity and rigor has also cost me dearly—it has meant that I lost time to insert my voice in public discourse and lost the opportunity to shape meaning-making regarding experiences related to the Black community. I have lost time in trying to appeal to authority figures who enact their power within the classroom and beyond by being passive in how disconnected "top" scholarship was to my experiences and others similar to me. However, being in these spaces and speaking upon these issues is a great privilege and one that comes with great responsibility. Without dissent, systems will never change. As I learn and grow, I aim to defy expectations and push back on hegemonic systems through my voice, which begins by sharing my personal experiences. Autoethnography offers me space to add my own voice and experiences to academic discourse. Through autoethnography and personal narratives, we are enacting agency to tell our own stories and reflect on our personal experiences. While we engage in self-disclosure and immerse our writing in our own real-life experiences, we invite our readers to walk along this journey with us. Audiences are also encouraged to engage in self-reflection regarding the topic(s) discussed in hopes that they will reach some personal level of growth upon completion of the reading. Further, personal narratives are most potent for connecting directly to the experiences shared. As the authors such as Cottom (2018) walked through their personal experiences, I was also walking through my own. I saw my life reflected upon theirs. I want my chapter to do the same for readers.

Based on my research and personal experiences, there are three general interrelations between race/racial discrimination and a Black person's mental health. First, racism directly affects the mental health of Black people when they experience it firsthand, both overtly and covertly. For instance, Black people often experience racial battle fatigue due to constantly fighting race-based discrimination, which leads to anxiety, mood swings, high blood pressure, and other health outcomes (Smith, Yosso, & Solórzano, 2011). Second, racism indirectly affects mental health as racial discrimination is often positively related to other societal inequities such as economic, educational, and political inequities and lack of representation and support (Bailey et al., 2017; Economic Policy Institute, 2019). Indirect racism also includes exposure of racism imposed onto other Black persons, such as police brutality witnessed in the media. Third, race and racial discrimination impact help-seeking behaviors around mental health concerns within Black communities (Avent, Cashwell, & Brown-Jeffy, 2013; Snowden, 2001). While each of these correlations is between race/racism and Black mental health, the third correlation connects the first two as direct and indirect racism affect help-seeking behaviors.

My chapter explores each of these perspectives of mental health in the Black community through the lens of my own experiences and organized around the following themes: racial trauma; stigma; mistrust of mainstream health and medical services; and lack of access to care. I end with a call to action and with a final note on my own healing journey to inspire readers to do the work to heal themselves and work on behalf of better mental health outcomes for the Black community.

In sharing my experiences, I am not under the illusion that Black people, Black women, or even Black women who identify as gay lead monolithic lives. Instead, my narrative serves to share a reality from my social location to build a more holistic and truthful narrative of mental health. I use my unique position as a critical interpretive researcher alongside autoethnographic methods to intertwine my experiences with existing literature and build upon theory. As a scholar, I believe that all research serves a purpose. We either implicitly perpetuate systems of power or work to expose them through our research. Within each section of this chapter, some form of power will be exposed in efforts to ultimately work towards more health equity for the Black community. It is important to note that none of these hegemonic systems of power are profoundly new, although my experiences are original to me specifically. I must pay homage to those before me who have gone to great lengths to ensure scholars such as myself have knowledge to build upon and work to continue. I hope that this chapter continues to expand space for other Black people to share their stories and expose systems of power and insalubrious mindsets.

Black Mental Health

Black people underutilize mental health services. Yet, Black people are more frequently diagnosed with major mental illnesses, more frequently *mis*diagnosed with mental illness, less frequently diagnosed with mood disorders, less likely to be offered evidence-based medication or psychotherapy, less frequently included in research, most likely to be incarcerated with mental health conditions, have lower rates of mental health service use, and often receive poorer quality of care (American Psychiatric Association, 2017). These health outcomes are due to a history of societal, economic, and political inequalities which have led to further barriers discouraging Black people from seeking the assistance needed to manage their mental health. Moreover, these barriers have led to unhealthy coping behaviors within Black communities. For Black individuals to truly begin healing and consider healthier mental health practices, we must begin to break down barriers that are causing blockages within the community. The first step to alleviating these barriers is to promote awareness and be intentional regarding the issues that need to be addressed.

Research supports that race and racial discrimination should be highlighted as important factors in understanding mental health within Black communities (Conner et al., 2010; Fischer & Shaw, 1999; Porter, 2018; Williams, 2018). Throughout this analysis, I will cover racial trauma, stigma, mistrust, and lack of access as barriers to seeking mental health assistance. Each barrier will be situated in race as a Black person's identity is inseparable from these barriers.

Race is an imperative concept in identifying, understanding, and dismantling barriers to care and shifting the overall narrative around mental health. There are norms within Black communities that must be addressed as well as discriminatory practices imposed onto Black communities that must be changed. Each of the three interrelations discussed above (that racism directly affects mental health; that racism indirectly affects mental health; and that both direct and indirect racism interfere with help-seeking) must all be addressed within the context of barriers that exist within Black communities themselves. We all have work to do, and we all have a role to play.

Racial Trauma and Racism

> I ran down to my best friend's house, eager to play. We always played together after school and on the weekends. To me, this day was no different, until I met her outside. My friend had a new friend. It was exciting. We all could play together. My excitement was halted when my friend told me that she did not want to play with me today, only with her new friend. Confused, I asked why. They both laughed, looked at me, and told me I was different. I asked her how. She replied that I was just different, and they were more alike. Her new friend said, "Yeah, look at our hair". The difference was that I was Black; my best friend, and her new friend, were White. Since then, subconsciously, I always sought out a Black friend.

I can recall many personal experiences of racism, such as being outcasted, called the n-word, criminally stereotyped, experiencing Blackface, and being physically threatened for even teaching equality as a Black instructor. Yet, those are not the experiences that affect me the most. I like to think I have somewhat "thick skin" regarding the pain inflicted upon me. Much more than my own direct experiences with racism, though, the trauma inflicted upon my family and our youth by virtue of direct racism burden me and affect my mental well-being to the highest degree. The stories of discrimination and oppression my family had to endure is devastating—heartbreaking. I am burdened thinking about how we were not allowed nourishment in certain establishments because "coloreds" were not allowed. Yes, we, including me—instances such as this happened while I was a child. How the only work available for my family was to do chores in White houses for pennies on the dollar. How my grandfather's comments in classes were degraded, but when a White woman shared those same sentiments, she was praised. What hurts even more as an academic is that such stories are being muted. Every lesson I had on slavery in grade school was whitewashed and framed as if it were some lapse in judgment at one small moment of time. It is clear that some would rather erase the "stain" of slavery; to momentarily appease us, they teach some rewritten fraction of the same story. There was always this disconnect between slavery and myself, as a Black person, in my history lessons. The pain and generational connection became real when I stopped viewing them as slaves, but as my family. Slavery is not some mark in the past that can be forgotten as its effects are very much still alive today. While I am optimistic of a greater future for my Black son, history has a way of repeating itself.

Many people experience inequalities regardless of race or ethnicity such as economic hardships, educational malpractice, housing indignities, occupational mortifications, and more. Black communities often experience these inequalities in addition to, and often as a result of, racism. Racism is real. Race is a social concept historically ingrained within our society that has caused great systematic oppression and discrimination to communities of color (Smith, 2014; Washington, 2008). Although racism is a concept that many people avoid due to the uncomfortable nature of discourse and facing reality, it is a foundational aspect of the specific trauma often experienced by Black people. Therefore, it is not one that can be ignored or forgotten (Fernando, 2010).

People often believe that if racism is not overt, then it does not exist. In actuality, indirect forms of racism such as covert racism, vicarious racism, and microaggressions are just as traumatic. The constant battle of deflecting racism and determining the safest and most effective ways to navigate white spaces is emotionally, mentally, and physically draining (Smith, 2014). This is a battle that Black people often encounter daily; it leads to things like racial PTSD and Racial Battle Fatigue. When we repeatedly experience traumatic events, our bodies begin to keep a recollection of those instances as we learn which actions lead to the most desirable outcomes (Menakem, 2017). The fatigue we experience may be our bodies signaling we need rest (Rowe, 2020). However, our family members were not afforded many opportunities to rest. Regardless of any battles that were encountered, they had to keep going, to keep fighting to live. This lack of space to rest, to take care of ourselves, led to an innate sense of strength within the Black community. Consequently, we suppress and deny when we may need help. This frame is quite logical when the only professional help available is from those you feel you cannot trust; those who've, throughout history, created conditions where such rest and care were impossible. It is a history of prejudice, mistreatment, abuse, neglect, and discrimination. As a result, alternative coping ways were developed, which have been more harmful in the long run.

Today, many of us keep this fight going by increasing awareness regarding alternative healing methods to provide our future generations with healthier means of understanding, dealing with, and sharing their emotions. For instance, regarding the vignette above, I suppressed that memory for ten years. I never told anyone. My way of fixing the problem was to avoid the possibility that situations like that one could occur again by actively seeking Black friends.

Therefore, I did not allow myself to have close White friends. Many within my community have utilized this coping mechanism of avoidance. Many also realize how emotionally damaging that may have been—to remain mute regarding trauma. Avenues, such as therapy, are now being normalized as ways to heal and work through such racial trauma before the fatigue hits. However, stigma related to mental health in the Black community also leads to a culture of silence around mental health struggles. I want my story to interrupt that silence and encourage others to do the same.

Stigma as a Barrier to Help-Seeking

I grew up learning concepts we should and should not talk about—mental health being one of them. As children, we are like sponges. We get fed information and take it in as truth. These truths are either reinforced or challenged as we continue to grow and encounter other experiences. I honestly do not have a vast recollection of conversations surrounding mental health specifically. I do not remember the word "health" being associated with "mental." However, when someone acted differently in a way that I did not quite understand, I do remember hearing messages such as "they're just crazy," "they have mental issues," and "we're going to pray about it." So, if someone was having issues that were not explained physically, I just assumed they were "crazy." I was taught not to ever talk about anyone and to mind my business. Still, I can admit that I did not understand them; therefore, I was not open to the idea that I may one day experience some of those emotions myself.

It took me 24 years to accept that everyone has mental health—everyone experiences some form of mental distress throughout their lifetime. However, I did not realize getting help for these concerns was just as normal as getting help for physical concerns. I had to hit rock bottom before I even considered seeking assistance. Prior to reaching my limit, I kept everything in. I never asked for help. I was afraid to voice my emotions, to speak up for myself, and to have difficult conversations. I became a people pleaser. I did not want to be perceived as weak. I tried to fix everything on my own and to make everyone else happy. All the traumatic experiences in my life piled up as I never talked about or acknowledged them. I thought I was strong for pushing past them, but I never healed. While I thought I was doing what was best, my suppression was harming my personal health and relationships. It was not until I sought professional help that this all became clear. My reluctance to seek help was undoubtedly related to stigma.

Stigma is one of the largest barriers impeding people from seeking mental health assistance. Mental illness is a highly stigmatized concept by the general public as it is one of the least accepted illnesses (Bharadwaj, Pai, & Suziedelyte, 2017; Corrigan, 2000; Hinshaw, 2007). Stigma occurs when society exposes something as unusual or deviant from the norm to discount, discredit, or taint

(Goffman, 2016). When something is stigmatized, it becomes less desirable so that a person might maintain a certain social status by avoiding such discreditation. Although an attribute or behavior may be socially less desirable, the attribute may still exist within people. When one realizes that an attribute they possess is stigmatized, they typically attempt to conceal it, and this prevents people from seeking assistance (Bharadwaj, Pai, & Suziedelyte, 2017). While mental health stigma exists in the general population, additional stigma also exists within Black communities, which further discourages Black people from seeking professional support.

Mental health stigma is prevalent within the Black community as needing mental health care is seen as a sign of weakness. Culturally, Black people are expected to be strong and resilient (Samuel, 2019). When a person shows signs of mental distress or illness, it is either equated with being weak or "crazy". For instance, Kyaien O. Conner et al. (2010) found that when their participants disclosed their mental health experiences, they would experience stereotyping and discrimination from within the Black community. People would see a person as "crazy," and this stigmatization led many people to hide their mental illnesses to avoid that moniker. Moreover, support was nonexistent for those who sought help, leading to Black community members denying that they had an illness. In the same study, it was found that some participants suppressed their emotions so much that they were in denial about the fact that they might have been depressed. The participants explained that they would stay busy, making it easier for them to forget about their mental illness (Conner et al., 2010).

It is typical to think of stigma in relation to the individual experiencing mental health distress. However, stigma is also a factor in how we as family, friends, and community members may interfere in helping someone else seek assistance. Velma Murry et al. (2011) conducted a study on the families of adolescents and found that Black mothers were afraid to seek mental health assistance for their children due to fear of being judged by their communities. The mothers were not only fearful of their children being judged, but they were also afraid of being judged themselves; indeed, children are often considered reflections of their parents. There are, thus, times when it is possible to inadvertently (explicitly and implicitly) discourage people from helping others with mental health concerns due to stigma. Stigma related to mental health can also prevent us from reaching out to people and lending a helping hand.

While considerable stigma exists within Black communities, stereotypes about Black people and mental health are created and/or reinforced outside of the community, and these stereotypes further strengthen that stigma. Studies show, for example, that the media reinforces stigma surrounding mental health and Black people; one implicit reinforcement of stigma is a lack of representation surrounding Black people and mental health assistance. Likewise, in Conner et al.'s (2010) study mentioned above, participants also reported that they only saw White people on mental health advertisements, which communicated that mental health services were for White people. Thus, lack of representation communicates that a particular attribute, experience, or service is only for those represented. Representations of mental health help-seeking as a White activity implicitly discourages Black people from seeking assistance, and when they are looking for ways to manage their mental health, professional treatment is too often considered a last resort. Beyond stigma, members of the Black community are also reluctant to seek out help for mental health concerns due to a very reasonable mistrust of mainstream health and medical services stemming from healthcare's history of abusing Black bodies.

Mistrust of Mainstream Health and Medical Services

> I received many lectures from my Grandmother on why we should not trust the White man. Somehow, I automatically knew the White man meant the larger community and those in power. We always went to my Granny's house and hung out with her, watching soap operas. She always gave us advice, not only as her grandchildren, but as her Black grandchildren. It seemed random at the time. I understood what she was saying, I was just too young to understand the impact. One thing she always told us was to not get caught up in the system, criminally or medically. We could not trust the White man because [they] never had our best interests at heart. She never wanted us to be naïve or manipulated. We had a remedy for everything, until we didn't.

As I began to accept therapy as a viable option for understanding and healing, I began researching everything I could about therapy. I listened to podcasts such as Between Sessions, read books similar to those referenced here, and listened to other people's experiences. A common theme amongst them was the importance of a cultural understanding between a client and their therapist. In other words, Black clients felt safer and more understood by Black therapists. Black women felt safer and more understood with Black women therapists. This is not to say that therapists of other races and ethnicities do not work for Black people. Some may, but for me, this led me to only trusting a Black woman therapist.

I did not reach my decision to only find a Black woman therapist solely from my research; my personal experiences played a vital role as well. I have been the first or the only Black woman in a room too often. In those spaces, I have been tokenized and viewed as the spokesperson. I have often served as a teacher to my teachers and peers. Material often discussed in my classes was not representative of my people. Everything was illustrative of White experiences and perspectives. Therefore, whenever I shared a different perspective and my own experiences, I had to justify my standpoint as a Black woman because no one else in the room understood. No one else in the room experienced life as a

Black woman. It was a demeaning, draining, and exhausting experience every time. I did not want to experience the same thing with my therapist. I did not want to unpack some of the most traumatic experiences in my life and have to explain why they were traumatic. I did not want to teach my therapist things they may not have understood culturally. My personal experiences taught me that much.

Health professionals are often viewed as untrustworthy in Black communities, at least in those I was immersed in as per the vignette above. In addition to the lack of cultural understanding, others are also apprehensive regarding the motives behind formal assistance in health-related issues due to the history of unethical research studies in the medical field. The Tuskegee experiment, unethical testing and sharing of Henrietta Lacks' cells and medical information without consent, experiments on Black women without anesthesia or medical ethicists or consent to improve the reproductive health of White women, stealing of enslaved bodies after death for experiments…the list of unethical medical practices goes on and on. These historical studies and practices cause apprehension within the Black community of trusting medical professionals, more specifically White medical professionals, who make up most of the medical fields. Moreover, these stories are often muted as many White professionals do not learn such studies were conducted.

It is imperative for all medical professionals to learn of these unethical studies because they shift narratives and start the conversation on how to minimize the effects of these studies in the present. As stated, mainstream American medicine was built to benefit White people. The tests, diagnoses, symptoms, and treatments were all developed based on and for White people. Thus, the foundation of health and medicine in the United States privileges White people at the expense of those whose symptoms or treatment options may be different. Consequently, if someone's symptoms of a disease are different than that of White people's, then it most often goes undiagnosed or mistreated. Further, the medical field has underlying assumptions about Black people, such as the belief that Black people have a higher pain tolerance than White people (Byrne et al., 2015). This erroneous belief leads to a lack of urgency in care for Black patients, which could be deadly. There are endless stories of Black people experiencing some form of conscious or subconscious prejudice or discrimination in health and medical settings, so it is not surprising that they respond by avoiding care.

When I was younger, I frequently experienced sharp pains in my chest accompanied by difficulty in breathing. My parents took me to the doctor. I received an EKG. I had a bit of an enlarged heart, but other than that nothing was wrong. When the sharp pains persisted, we assumed it was asthma. As a high-performing athlete, it did not add up. I was then diagnosed with stress-induced asthma. I was unsure of what that meant, other than the fact that I had a really hard time breathing during moments of high stress. I received a pump and used it for a while, but eventually taught myself to calm down and catch my breath whenever my chest started to contract. Reflecting back, this is the time I started struggling with my sexuality, though I did not make the connection at the time. While I was able to develop these coping mechanisms on my own, it is clear that I could have benefited from targeted mental health help, such as talk therapy or behavior modification, yet it was not offered.

Concerning mental health specifically, some argue that mental health professionals do not really care about helping Black people. Instead, mental health professionals just prescribe medicine without the proper assessment of one's mental state or without trying less invasive forms of treatment such as therapy or counseling (Conner et al., 2010). This move to medication without exploring other options is problematic as the medication-first approach too often stems from prejudicial and stereotypical preconceptions about therapy as not for Black people. Further, this mistrust results in many Black people consulting doctors reactively rather than proactively—they seek out help only when the problem becomes so significant that it can no longer be ignored. This is a form of systematic racism. Even when Black people do want to seek help, they cannot always access quality care.

Lack of Access

After I began therapy, I became an avid advocate for mental health within Black communities. Around that time, I was engaged in a conversation regarding my experiences in an attempt to shift stigma and encourage another to try therapy. It worked—they were open to the idea of therapy as a proactive measure. They were ready to be vulnerable and understand their emotions to truly heal. Still, they were unable to go. I remember, at the end of our conversation, they stated,

"I mean that's nice, but I can't afford that."

Black communities have a high risk of having little to no access to mental health treatment. Regarding insurance, Black people are very likely to be covered by Medicaid or uninsured (Wells et al., 2001). While Medicaid offsets some medical costs like other forms of insurance and is designed to help underserved populations and to minimize disparities, it does not offer coverage for mental health services to the degree that regular insurance or wealth might. Medicaid covers 21% of the population, and 33% of the population covered are Black (KFF, n.d.). While Black people make up 13.4% of the population (Census Bureau, 2019), they account for over a third of the population covered by Medicaid. Thus, a significant number of Black people in need of assistance have little to no access to adequate healthcare.

Many Black families are also unable to seek treatment because of financial strain. Some families cannot afford adequate treatment financially; some are unable to get time off from work to attend mental health appointments. Others are unable to physically travel to facilities (Chow, Jaffee, & Snowden, 2003; Murry et al., 2011; Ward, Clark, & Heidrich, 2009). Just as Medicaid does not always offset the entire cost of medical expenses, it also does not account for travel expenses. Many families live far from professional mental health facilities. Moreover, Black families who live in rural and urban areas are both highly affected by mental health issues. For instance, Susan Busch and Colleen Barry (2007) found that mental illnesses such as depression, ADD, and anxiety are shown to be most prevalent among children who reside in rural areas, while Nicholas Ialongo et al. (2004) also found that major depressive disorder was most prevalent among young Black people who lived in urban areas. However, only 10% of those who were identified as experiencing or have experienced major depressive disorder received any professional assistance. Ultimately, there is a lack of resources to bridge the gap in mental health inequities.

Call to Action and Directions for Future Research

As Rheeda Walker (2020) explained,

> In the Black community, very few people feel that they have someone reliable and trustworthy to call. As a result, the interplay of stigma, limited knowledge, unexpressed pain, and lack of access conspires to keep many families from overcoming unnecessary cycles of hurt. It is time for a shift. It is time to have more honest conversations. If you are going to reinforce your mind, we are going to have to be honest about the problem at hand.
> *(p. 17)*

As Walker makes clear, mental health is a complex concept to address; coupled with systematic inequities, it becomes much more complicated. We all play a part in working toward a more health equitable society, both within and outside Black communities. As researchers and practitioners, we are responsible for ensuring a psychologically and physically safe and equitable health environment for everyone and for providing culturally fit resources when needed. As community members, we have a responsibility to provide healthy alternatives of healing and open, inclusive perspectives on mental health in hopes of decreasing the trauma future generations might endure. Below is a call to action for both researchers and community members.

First, future researchers should continue to examine the intricacies of the mental health of Black people to dismantle systems of oppression that create barriers to care and to rebuild more equitable and culturally fit programs and trainings. To this end, future work in mental health rhetoric should conduct community-based participatory research to understand first-hand experiences further and identify ways to decrease inequities. It is important to continue to archive and share stories to raise awareness of experiences and work toward change. These stories must come from community members, and identified changes should be based on collaborative work with community researchers.

As well, certain organizations have begun implementing changes to address inequities; thus, future research should be conducted to determine the efficacy of such changes from a culturally centered perspective, such as the approach discussed in Lisa DeTora and Tomeka Robinson's chapter in this volume. Similar to community-based participatory research, community members must be included in changes implemented following inquiries into how organizational efforts are or are not impacting inequities as these community members are affected.

Importantly, Black researchers are already doing much of this work. However, their voices and studies as researchers are being muted and overlooked. I hope readers will educate themselves such that they are able to identify key scholars and research studies in this area, add these studies to their personal reference lists, publish them in top journals and books, include them in their syllabi, and insert them in discussions and conferences. Several representative works are cited in this chapter, which could offer a starting point.

As community members, readers might identify ways they can personally work toward healing. Oftentimes, we deal with such issues as trauma and mental health struggles through religion, self-concealment, or informal social support. This is not a call to completely revamp these ways of coping, but instead a call to refine and add to current practices to shift from coping to healing. Religion is a great source of strength and support; praying could be used in addition to other more concrete forms of healing. I am still a firm believer in protecting your personal business. However, too much self-concealment can be self-destructive. We must determine when and what we should speak up about to protect our mental well-being while also creating and maintaining boundaries.

When trust is an issue, we often rely on informal forms of social support such as through our family, friends, and significant others. These people should be safe spaces in which we can confide. Still, we must be careful to not treat them as therapists. There are many times when trauma is reoccurring and deeply rooted, and we need more tools for understanding and shifting behavior; these are often found in clinical mental health contexts. Our informal peers are unable to perform these actions for us. Instead, there are times in which we should seek the counsel of a therapist. From my own experience, I can say with confidence that only you can determine what you need and when you need it. Practice listening to your body and subconscious mind as it often signals when we need assistance.

I also want to encourage others to continue to share their stories. Stories and narratives are powerful. They embody a certain level of transparency; they allow others to relate and to empathize. They provide implications and prescriptions for ways people can approach their own experiences. Your story may be the deciding factor for someone to become more aware, feel heard, empowered, inspired, seek assistance, speak up. Stories not only connect us, but they also provide a vivid illustration of reality for those who have different experiences. You never know—but keep sharing.

Moreover, have conversations with your family, friends, and other community members. Normalize conversations around difficult topics, behaviors, emotions, and healing practices. Speak up when you may need assistance, be available (if you have the emotional capacity) for others, work on changing unhealthy habits within our families, encourage our children to express their feelings, and have routine check-ins.

Conclusion

It took me going through the perfect traumatic storm for me to even consider therapy. I had to experience a form of depression that I could not pull myself out of. I sought solace in those I was closest to, but that was not enough. I was constantly venting about my experiences and emotions without actually healing. I was mentally constrained within my own mind—repeating patterns, memories, and emotions. I was merely surviving. I knew what I needed to do to make it through each day, to appear happy. Still, at the end of each day, I was in pain. I knew how to put on a front in public while battling difficulties with eating, sleeping, working—basic everyday tasks. I knew how to survive. The goal is not to survive. The goal is to heal and live abundantly. I wanted to live. I wanted to experience joy. I wanted to exist with the option of choosing happiness. I wanted to be unburdened. I wanted to heal—not only to relieve myself of pain from my own trauma but also to be more cognizant of the trauma I inflict onto others. I wanted to learn how to mitigate pain on my own without suppression and avoidance. So, I took that first step. I went to therapy. It is the best decision I made.

Through therapy, I learned how to identify, explain, and work through difficulties and triggers. I have been able to connect my current behaviors to past experiences. Through these connections, I am able to confront the anchor holding me to the triggers and my behavior. Through confronting the actual experience, I am slowly able to detach and separate the past from the present, which allows me a greater mental capacity to truly be in the present moment. As I identify and work through my personal triggers, I learn different techniques for changing my behavior and thought process around those triggers to be more positive. As much as therapy has helped me to heal from my own trauma, it most importantly has provided me avenues and a mind frame for compassion, understanding, and patience. Truth is, we all will experience trauma and inflict trauma onto someone else. Once we understand ourselves and break connections to unhealthy practices and harmful experiences, we are able to become better people to others. That is what will lead to a freer and more equitable future.

Note to Leave You With

A lot of times when I share these experiences with people, I receive sympathy and apologies. This chapter is not written in search of an apology. This chapter is written to raise awareness. To check our own biases; to disrupt and dismantle a system that is inherently racist, discriminatory, and prejudice. To create a better and more equitable future for generations to come. To normalize healing through conversation. To use our voices to enact change within our larger society, community, and family. It starts and continues with you. Find your place, find your voice, heal yourself, and do the work.

Acknowledgments

This book chapter is by far one of the most difficult pieces I have written. Without the support of many people, this would not have been possible.

I have to start by thanking my amazing wife, Aleysha. Thank you for reading all my drafts, helping me to identify stories, helping me reflect, and pulling me through when I needed it. To my son Kingston, thank you for helping me analyze my experiences and allowing me time to work.

To my parents and grandparents, thank you so much for everything you have taught me and laying the foundation for me to become the woman I am today. Thank you so much for being vulnerable with me, sharing your experiences, and talking with me through mine.

To my sister and brother, thank you so much for all your support every step of the way and always being there when I needed. I worked through so many of these stories with you, thank you.

To Goyland, thank you for allowing me to read through this chapter with you. You provided me with much knowledge, motivation, and guidance.

Lastly, Cathryn and Lisa, thank you so much for all your patience, understanding, and great guidance. You have supported me with open arms the whole way. Thank you.

References

American Psychiatric Association. (2017). *Mental health disparities: African Americans.* American Psychiatric Association.

Avent, Janeé R., Cashwell, Craig S., & Brown-Jeffy, Shelly. (2015). African American pastors on mental health, coping, and help-seeking. *Counseling and Values, 60*(1), 32–47. https://doi.org/10.1002/j.2161-007X.2015.00059.x

Bailey, Zinzi D., Krieger, Nancy, Agénor, Madina, Graves, Jasmine, Linos, Natalina, & Bassett, Mary T. (2017). Structural racism and health inequities in the USA: evidence and interventions. *The Lancet, 389*(10077), 1453–1463. https://doi.org/10.1016/S0140-6736(17)30569-X

Bharadwaj, Prashant, Pai, Mallesh M., & Suziedelyte, Agne. (2017). Mental health stigma. *Economics Letters, 159*(C), 57–60. doi:10.1016/j.econlet.2017.06.028

Busch, Susan H., & Barry, Colleen L. (2007). Mental health disorders in childhood: Assessing the burden on families. *Health Affairs, 26*(4), 1088–1095. https://doi.org/10.1377/hlthaff.26.4.1088

Byrne, Michelle, Callahan, Barbara, Carlson, Karen, Daley, Linda, Magorian, Kathy, Phillips, Pamela, & Wilhelm, Sue. (2015). *Nursing: A concept-based approach to learning volume I, I, III.* Pearson Education.

Census Bureau. (2019, July 1). *Quick fact United States.* United States Census Bureau.

Chow, Julian. C. C., Jaffee, Kim, & Snowden, Lonnie. (2003). Racial/ethnic disparities in the use of mental health services in poverty areas. *American Journal of Public Health, 93*(5), 792–797. doi:10.2105/ajph.93.5.792

Conner, Kyaien O., Lee, Brenda, Mayers, Vanessa, Robinson, Deborah, Reynolds III, Charles F., Albert, Steve, & Brown, Charlotte. (2010). Attitudes and beliefs about mental health among African American older adults suffering from depression. *Journal of Aging Studies, 24*(4), 266–277. doi:10.1016/j.jaging.2010.05.007

Corrigan, Patrick. W. (2000). Mental health stigma as social attribution: Implications for research methods and attitude change. *Clinical Psychology: Science and Practice, 7*(1), 48–67. https://doi.org/10.1093/clipsy.7.1.48

Cottom, Tressie M. (2018). *Thick: and other essays.* The New Press.

Curthoys, Ann, & McGrath, Ann. (2011). How to avoid writer's block. In Ann Curthoys & Ann McGrath (Eds.), *How to write history that people want to read* (pp. 101–116). Palgrave Macmillan.

Delgado, Richard, & Stefancic, Jean. (2017). *Critical race theory: An introduction* (Vol. 20). NYU Press.

Fernando, Suman. (2010). *Mental health, race and culture.* Macmillan International Higher Education.

Fischer, Ann R., & Shaw, Christina M. (1999). African Americans' mental health and perceptions of racist discrimination: The moderating effects of racial socialization experiences and self-esteem. *Journal of Counseling Psychology, 46*(3), 395–407.

Goffman, Erving. (2016). Selections from stigma. In Lennard J. Davis (Ed.), *The disability studies reader,* 5th edition (pp. 133–134). Routledge.

Hinshaw, Stephen P. (2007): *The mark of shame: Stigma of mental illness and agenda for change.* Oxford University Press.

Ialongo, Nicholas, McCreary, Beth K., Pearson, Jane L., Koenig, Amy L., Schmidt, Norman B., Poduska, Jeanne, & Kellam, Sheppartd G. (2004). Major depressive disorder in a population of urban, African-American young adults: Prevalence, correlates, comorbidity and unmet mental health service need. *Journal of Affective Disorders, 79*(1–3), 127–136. doi:10.1016/S0165-0327(02)00456-1

KFF. (n.d.). *Medicaid coverage rates for the nonelderly by race/ethnicity.* Kaiser Family Foundation.

Lee, Sy-ying. (2005). The robustness of extensive reading: Evidence from two studies. *The International Journal of Foreign Language Teaching, 1*(3), 13–19.

Menakem, Resmaa. (2017). *My grandmother's hands: Racialized trauma and the pathway to mending our hearts and bodies.* Central Recovery Press.

Murry, Velma M., Heflinger, Craig A., Suiter, Sarah V., & Brody, Gene H. (2011). Examining perceptions about mental health care and help-seeking among rural African American families of adolescents. *Journal of Youth and Adolescence, 40*(9), 1118–1131. doi:10.1007/s10964-010-9627-1

Phillips, Rasheedah, Picot, Iresha, & Hazzard, Vanessa. (2015). *The color of hope: People of color mental health narratives.* CreateSpace Independent Publishing Platform.

Porter, Jeannette. (2018). *In the pastor's study: A grounded theory analysis of African American Baptist ministers' communication on mental health and illness.* [Doctoral dissertation, UNC]. doi:10.17615/dpn9-3m78

Rowe, Sheila W. (2020) *Healing racial trauma: The road to resilience.* IVP Books.

Samuel, Melody. (2019). *Mental health concerns in African American churches: Pastoral preparedness in counseling.* [Master's thesis, Gardner-Webb University].

Smith, William. A. (2014). *Racial battle fatigue in higher education: Exposing the myth of post-racial America.* Rowman & Littlefield.

Smith, William A., Yosso, Tara J., & Solórzano, Daniel G. (2011). Challenging racial battle fatigue on historically White campuses: A critical race examination of race-related stress. In Rodney D. Coates (Ed.), *Covert racism* (pp. 211–237). BRILL.

Snowden, Lonnie R. (2001). Barriers to effective mental health services for African Americans. *Mental Health Services Research, 3*(4), 181–187. doi:10.1023/a:1013172913880

Walker, Rheeda. (2020). The unapologetic guide to black mental health: Navigate an unequal system, learn tools for emotional wellness, and get the help you deserve. *New Harbinger Publications.*

Ward, Earlise C., Clark, Le Ondra., & Heidrich, Susan (2009). African American women's beliefs, coping behaviors, and barriers to seeking mental health services. *Qualitative Health Research, 19*(11), 1589–1601. doi:10.1177/1049732309350686

Washington, Harriet A. (2008). *Medical apartheid: The dark history of medical experimentation on black Americans from colonial times to present.* Anchor.

Wells, Kenneth, Klap, Ruth, Koike, Alan, & Sherbourne, Cathy. (2001). Ethnic disparities in unmet need for alcoholism, drug abuse, and mental health care. *American Journal of Psychiatry, 158*(12), 2027–2032. doi:10.1176/appi.ajp.158.12.2027

Williams, David R. (2018). Stress and the mental health of populations of color: Advancing our understanding of race-related stressors. *Journal of Health and Social Behavior, 59*(4), 466–485. doi:10.1177/0022146518814251

Williams, Jhacova, & Wilson, Valerie. (2019, August 27). *Black workers endure persistent racial disparities in employment outcomes.* Economic Policy Institute.

9

AN AUTOETHNOGRAPHIC EXAMINATION OF ANOSOGNOSIA IN A SIBLING EXHIBITING SEVERE PSYCHOSIS

Reimagining Inclusiveness in MHRR

Cynthia Ryan

Introduction

November 16, 2017. *Like many nights during the final nine months I spent with Dad, he and I sit side by side flipping the channels after dinner.*

The Magnificent Seven *is starting on* Classic Western Station. *We stick with this option, settling in for the predictable action and satisfying ending.*

"I'll never understand how we got here," Dad muttered in my direction.

"Got where?" I asked, grateful for a distraction from the shoot 'em up scene I'd seen a minimum of five times in recent memory.

"Your idiot brother," he said, shaking his head and smacking his lips to show his disgust. "One minute, you're holding a baby in your arms. The next, he has a record."

My father died two months following this exchange, lacking answers to the questions that all of us who've encountered Joe ask. Why did my brother abuse people and animals starting at a young age, laughing as they cried or fled in fear? How could he insist that he'd never done anything wrong and that there was "nothing the matter with him" after multiple incarcerations and court-mandated stays in psychiatric hospitals? What prevented Joe from forging a life, however imperfect, in which some relationships remain intact and his basic needs are met?

As a rhetoric of health and medicine (RHM) scholar, I recognize both the rhetorical complexity behind these questions and the thorny implication of any potential answers, whether provided by medical experts or through collective soul-searching. It's difficult to imagine that any answers, too, will remedy years of self- and other-inflicted pain. Still, I find myself grasping for fragments of understanding that require reckoning with Joe's mental illness and the many episodes with Joe that have constituted a significant part of my life during the

DOI: 10.4324/9781003144854-12

past five-plus decades. Evidence of my only sibling's psychosis is plentiful. Now in his sixties, Joe's decline into chaos has hastened at the same time that it falls on me to keep tabs on my brother's whereabouts and to help myriad people within different health and legal systems grapple with the visible ramifications of Joe's illness. When his psychosis rages to the point of threatening to kill me and my family, it also falls on me to keep us all safe.

While mental health rhetoric research (MHRR) scholarship has addressed the marginalizing assumptions and problematic histories reflecting the treatment of those considered mentally ill, it has largely ignored examinations of individuals who exhibit what E. Fuller Torrey (2012) calls "anosognosia," meaning a "lack of [self] knowledge of disease" (p. 114). The condition of anosognosia, first associated with patients experiencing amputation of an appendage or paralysis following a stroke, leads "affected individuals" to "deny their deficits and make up stories—called confabulations—to explain their disability" (p. 114). While Torrey admits that the number of individuals with severe psychosis who are unaware of their illness is relatively low, he also emphasizes that this population is by far the most dangerous. Since their denial of illness often leads them to refuse medications and other treatments, they are more likely to act in ways that, in common parlance, endanger themselves and others. Such severe cases are also exacerbated by comorbidities, such as substance use disorders. Joe's extensive history of drug overdoses and violence against others is a case in point.

In addition to having intimate knowledge of how anosognosia complicates severe cases of chronic psychosis, I posit that members of this population may also be limited in their ability to engage rhetorically. For example, in his interactions with others, my brother consistently demonstrates an absence of what Diane Davis (2010) called "originary (or preoriginary) rhetoricity," specifically "an affect*ability* or persuad*ability*" necessary for "symbolic interaction" (p. 2, emphasis included in original). Importantly, too, the possibility that rhetoricity may be (dis)*ab[led]* wholly or partially in cases of severe psychosis accompanied by anosognosia complicates the notion in MHRR and in disability studies that stigma surrounding mental illness might be deflected via interrogating what it means to be "normal" or "abnormal" in society and/or by inviting in the voices of those displaying unconventional behaviors associated with cognitive disorders—solutions that do make good sense when considered in light of most cases of mental illness, yet are not at all applicable to cases where a person is truly a danger to themselves and to others. Individuals showing signs of anosognosia alongside severe psychosis lack sufficient awareness of their behaviors, and the effects of those behaviors in a larger social context, to participate "ethically" and "safely" in rhetorical exchanges. As I reveal in this chapter, textual evidence drawn from documented conversations with Joe reveals features of what Jenell Johnson (2010) referred to as *kakoethos* or "anti-*ethos*" associated with stigmatizing labels like "worthless, evil, dirty, ugly, weak, cowardly, envious, dangerous" (p. 465). Each of these labels has been hurled at my sibling, often in conjunction with egregious actions that Joe denies, including those that have been widely observed and/or documented. During his 61 years, Joe has been incarcerated in more than a dozen states for crimes including armed robbery, drug trafficking, sexual assault, and illegal possession of weapons. Following such offenses, he has been committed multiple times to psychiatric institutions and drug and alcohol rehabilitation centers, all reflecting the "recurring penal pilgrimages" that Torrey (2012) claimed are common among individuals suffering from severe psychosis, yet largely unaware of their illness (p. 55). These journeys in and out of what Erving Goffman (1961) called "total institutions" (p. 7) contribute to the derogatory characterization of those with mental illness diagnoses at the same time "curtailment of self" occurs in these environments as "inmates" attempt to survive (p. 14).

Joe frequently engages, perhaps unknowingly, in strategies reflecting *kakoethos* by boasting about antiethical actions as proof of his right-mindedness and the misjudgments of others, including family members, law enforcement, and psychiatrists. He brags about stealing items that have sentimental value to their rightful owners, following through on threats of sexual assault, carrying knives that he can wield against anyone who gets in his way, and burying three ex-wives who were addicted to drugs and alcohol. That is, in his estimation, his ability to carry out such things are signs of his superiority, yet bragging about these things only conveys poor character to most audiences. As such, it is difficult to characterize Joe's rhetorical capabilities.

MHRR scholars have, likewise, grappled with whether those with mental illness diagnoses can achieve rhetoricity. Drawing on the work of Katie Rose Guest Pryal (2010), Catherine Prendergast (2014) acknowledged that individuals exhibiting signs of mental illness who commit to a medication protocol may oftentimes reclaim rhetoricity, a revision of her previous claim that "to be disabled mentally is to be disabled rhetorically" (Prendergast, 2001, p. 57). But individuals with severe psychosis and anosognosia who, like my sibling, refuse to be treated for illnesses that they deny having can succumb to rhetorical exchanges that both further stigmatization and undercut attempts to display what Cathryn Molloy (2020) called "recuperative ethos" and "agile epistemologies" (pp. 122–124). That is, in cases of severe psychosis, it is unclear whether attempts to use rhetoric successfully get speakers any closer to their aims. In this chapter, I argue that new interventional spaces that acknowledge the unique material and discursive challenges witnessed in cases of severe psychosis accompanied by anosognosia are needed in MHRR. Even while I acknowledge it is a small group, ignoring this "subset" of the mentally ill population as well as the individuals affected by their thoughts and actions is to risk further marginalizing the most severely afflicted. This project, thus, answers Cathryn Molloy, Drew Holladay, and Lisa Melonçon's (2020) charge to further examine the "flexible boundaries" for the study of mental health through a rhetorical lens

(p. iv). By pushing out the boundary around what is usually discussed in relation to mental health and rhetoric, MHRR scholars may allow for cases of severe illness and attendant serious violence and destruction.

An Interpretive Performance Autoethnographic Approach

April 2021. Since Joe was released from the state hospital in Wyoming in early February 2021, a facility that houses an extensive psychiatric care unit, he has left more than 170 messages on my office phone, most recorded at night one right after another. Every few days, I download the messages and forward them to the police before clearing out my voicemail to make room for more recordings.

The nature of Joe's messages varies.

Joe recounts events from the past 60 years, accusing anyone who has "turned [their] backs on him" of small-mindedness, immorality, apathy, and destructive words and actions.

He demands money, a return call, a car. He's landed in a "nut house" or a jail, and it's my responsibility to help him out since "there's nothing wrong with [him]."

My brother describes in explicit detail violent acts, past and future. Vulgar accounts of his sexual abuse of me as a kid and of the women he's raped. He details the sequence of events that will unfold when he reaches my house in Birmingham and assaults me while I "whimper" helplessly. He engages in name-calling intended to reduce me to tears: "F——— C—t!"

As painful as the messages are, I worry when they stop coming. Those periods of silence spur anxiety because I don't know Joe's whereabouts. Has he been arrested or committed to a hospital? Is he lying in a morgue or en route to Birmingham?

Like my father, I ask myself how we got here. But really, I know. I've lived it one crisis at a time.

Following what Norman K. Denzin (2014) called "interpretive performance autoethnography," an approach which involves "tak[ing] up [a] person's life in its immediate particularity and … ground[ing] the life in its historical moment" (p. x), snapshots throughout this chapter document my experiences with a brother whose "interpersonal deficits" fall under the umbrella category of "antisocial personality disorder" according to the *DSM-V* (Cluster B, 301.7, F60.2) (American Psychiatric Association, 2013), specifically those behaviors associated with "psychopathy," "schizophrenia," and "bipolar II disorder." As I share fragments of "our" story from "my" perspective, I cast critical attention on the partiality of the account while drawing on the conventions of academic discourse, situating these experiences in existing MHRR reflecting the kind of multidisciplinary inquiry characteristic of the field of RHM as noted by Lisa Melançon and J. Blake Scott (2018). Undoubtedly, Joe would describe the moments I present differently. I recognize the ethical dilemma posed by offering this partial view while acknowledging that impartiality is impossible from either an epistemological or communicative perspective, yet I also acknowledge that this missing demographic in the MHRR literature is so vital to deepening conversations in the field that I am moving forward, however imperfectly, with this work.

There is no single moment that demonstrates what it's like to grow up with a brother who appears to lack a moral compass, no one memory that can encapsulate the deluge of emotions that emerge during any interaction with him. That said, theories of rhetorical ecologies help me to begin to articulate these things in terms of how they fit into MHRR. Building on the work of Steven Shaviro, Jenny Edbauer (2005) wrote that the "social field" from which rhetors draw in strategizing messages "is not comprised of discrete *sites* but from events that are shifting and moving, grafted onto and connected with other events" (p. 10). Edbauer urged a rethinking of rhetorical *situs*, environments conceptualized as "bordered, fixed-space location[s]," opting for an understanding of "public rhetorics (and rhetoric's publicness) as a circulating ecology of effects, enactments, and events" made possible by "shifting the lines of focus from *rhetorical situation* to *rhetorical ecologies*" (p. 9, emphasis in original). Such a construction broadens the perimeters for the kinds of questions that MHRR scholars ask as well as the fluidity of those questions over time. A "rhetorical ecologies" framework also better situates the lived experiences of individuals exhibiting signs of mental illness and those who dwell in their mutual environments. Rather than offering discrete components for examination and potential understanding—something that cosurvivors of individuals suffering from severe psychosis frequently seek—survivorship in this context is in constant flux, amid both the "private rhetorics" occurring behind closed doors and the "public rhetorics" that fuel these exchanges. As a case in point, I have struggled with how to chronicle the pain and suffering associated with Joe's mental illness that is both everywhere and nowhere in particular. I'm reminded of Christa Teston's (2017) claim that the "uncertainty posed by the ambiguous space between living and dying" becomes the province of science in a biomedical sphere, as authorities offer "medical evidence" to fill in the unknowns (p. 1). The "ambiguous space[s]" I share with my sibling are impossible to clarify by reference to positivist epistemologies, another reason for adopting an explicitly "ecological" (Edbauer, 2005) perspective grounded in an autoethnographic methodology as it makes room for families like mine.

Always. By the time I was five years old, I knew my brother was somebody who was not only willing, but eager, to hurt me. Every encounter we had was a negotiation.

"If you do x," he'd say, "then I won't throw this rock at your eye/make you let me touch you/shoot your cat/tell Mom what you got her for Christmas."

For the record, his promises were lies. Regardless of my acquiescence to his demands, Joe would throw the rock, touch me, shoot my pets, share my surprise gift just to cause me pain and assert his control. From my perspective as Joe's little sister, there were no real choices. At least nothing that might be considered a "win." Life with Joe was just plain exhausting.

Assumptions about Identity and Rhetoricity and Challenging Institutional Rhetorics in Current MHRR

July 2018. My youngest daughter and I are staying at the farmhouse in Illinois, beginning the first of many attempts to clear out the house in which my parents lived for more than 50 years following Dad's passing and Mom's relocation to a nursing home. Having recently learned of Dad's death, Joe is back in our hometown and enraged that he hadn't been notified. [For the record, I had tried to inform Joe of Dad's passing, but found it impossible to track him down as he traversed states and spent time in jails, rehab facilities, and homeless shelters.]

One night, as Helena and I slept, Joe appeared outside the kitchen window—the window now covered in bars and part of a highly-sensitive security system put in place for just this reason—and started banging and yelling: "I know you're in there, you b——-! Let me in or I'm gonna kill you!"

I called 911, waiting on the line for help to arrive. As Joe stood outside shaking the kitchen door and screaming to be let in that summer, I remained focused on the voice of the county dispatcher telling me how far away the deputies were from the house. The calming words spoken by an institutional representative, rather than the fiery threats spewed by my sibling, took precedent.

Joe was arrested that night (one of ten arrests during the following three weeks), and the next day Helena and I taped up the windows throughout the house to prevent Joe from peering inside as we armed ourselves with mace, crowbars, and aluminum baseball bats for the remainder of our stay.

Much scholarship in MHRR centers on the usurping of the voices of individuals diagnosed as mentally ill in favor of the seemingly more coherent talk of psychiatrists and others in positions of authority. As MHRR scholars have argued the need to dissolve the physical boundaries erected between the "mad" and those reflecting an ordered "moral" society, divisions exposed by many including Michel Foucault (1965), Roy Porter (2003), and Edward Shorter (1997), they have strived to honor the voices of the ostracized, past and present. Through presentations of the recovered narratives of asylum "inmates" (Goffman, 1961), scholars including Carol Berkenkotter (2008), Cristina Hanganu-Bresch and Carol Berkenkotter (2019), and Pamela Takayoshi (2020) offered a stark contrast to the case notes composed by clinicians whose job it was to justify the identities of the institutionalized as Other.

Turning to the modern landscape, Stephen P. Hinshaw (2007) asserted that since the development of the *DSM*, "statistical rarity" has become an ambiguous, yet pivotal, concept in labeling individuals as mentally ill (pp. 8–9), leading experts like Allen Frances (2013), a member of the task force for the *DSM-IV*, to argue that the medicalization of disorders considered "abnormal" has extended its reach in such a way that prevents most of society from claiming normality. MHRR scholars including Lucille Parkinson McCarthy (1991), J. Fred Reynolds, David C. Mair, and Pamela C. Fischer (1992) further complicate the clinical implications tied to the *DSM* as a rhetorically driven "charter document" (McCarthy, 1991) embedded in a biomedical perspective on psychiatry.

Demonstrating the reach of the *DSM* within a biomedical context, Kimberly K. Emmons (2008, 2014) showed that manufacturers of psychotropic medications also limit the identities that health consumers may adopt. Women, especially, are called to "self-doctor"/diagnose their emotional well-being through a "relatively two-dimensional representation of the language of illness" (p. 9). As Cynthia Lewiecki-Wilson (2003) noted, for individuals diagnosed with mental disability including mental retardation, "speech is … a problematic term," "creat[ing] a barrier excluding [these populations] not only from rhetoricity but also from full citizenship" (p. 158). Highlighting efforts to give voice to the silenced, N. Renuka Uthappa (2017) and Pryal (2010) provided evidence of increasing representation of the "rhetorically disabled" (Prendergast, 2001) in political and authorial spaces. The trajectory in MHRR is towards continued valuing of all identities, regardless of the labels associated with mental illness and disability, yet my own experiences lead me to believe that such work, while valuable, doesn't account for or include families like mine.

September 2020. During a conversation with a deputy at a county detention center in Wyoming, I learn that Joe either isn't cooperating or isn't capable of undergoing a psychiatric evaluation to assess his competency for standing trial. My brother refuses to answer the psychiatrist's questions and threatens to stab him and kill his children if he doesn't "f—leave" the room. It dawns on me that I never bothered to ask what Joe has done to land him in jail this time.

The judge orders that recordings from a surveillance camera inside Joe's cell be used as evidence in determining Joe's state of mind and whether he should stand trial or be sent to the state psychiatric hospital for further assessment and treatment.

"We've had people in here who've tried to drown their children," the deputy told me. "They've got nothing on your brother."

As Joe's next of kin and with his permission, I am contacted by the court-appointed psychiatrist for information about Joe's history. An assessment is eventually completed, and Joe is sent to the state hospital in Evanston, WY for the next few months.

No matter how many times I am enlisted to weigh in on situations related to Joe's actions, my gut is tied up in knots. I associate Joe with abuse, humiliation, threats to my physical and emotional well-being. But Joe is my only sibling and one of the last members of my family of origin. Should I attempt to help Joe escape the darkness—something that history has proven is unlikely to work—or do everything I can to ensure that he stays locked away and can't hurt anyone?

Despite its merits as I've outlined them above, missing from current MHRR is a consideration of the lived experience(s) associated with severe psychosis with anosognosia, both for individuals suffering from these disorders and for the cosurvivors who live alongside them. Given the rarity of occurrence, it is understandable that scholars often overlook this population or consider them a fiction constructed by the makers of popular horror movies. According to

Torrey (2012), the 2009 National Mental Health Information Center's estimates of "serious mental illness" was "12.8 million adults" (p. 5). Of this admittedly "imprecise" number,

> **5,000,000**: The number of individuals in the U.S. who have severe psychiatric disorders (schizophrenia, bipolar disorder with psychosis, depression with psychosis).
>
> **500,000:** The subset of the 4 million that is most problematic if not treated, estimated to be approximately 10 percent of the total. These are the individuals who are most often homeless, incarcerated, victimized, and/or violent. Most are not aware of their illness and do not take medication. Most of them need to be on some form of assisted treatment.
>
> **50,000:** The most overtly dangerous, 1 percent of the total. These individuals have been proven to be dangerous. They have committed violent acts and, if unmedicated, are likely to do so again. Most of them can live in the community as long as it is guaranteed that they are on medication to control their symptoms.
>
> *(pp. 5–6, emphasis in original)*

Drawing on my history with my sibling, Joe falls somewhere between the "500,000" and "50,000" subsets, increasingly meeting criteria for the population Torrey calls "the most overtly dangerous" (p. 6). By "assisted treatment," Torrey is referring to mandatory medication programs, whereby individuals who refuse treatment for severe psychosis because the presence of anosognosia makes them unaware of their illness submit to required surveillance and are restricted from certain governmental benefits (e.g., disability checks) unless they can prove compliance. From the perspective of MHRR, such a response seems like a significant step backwards—a rejection of the notion that diagnostic labels for mental illnesses are often more indicative of rhetorical responses to social values than identifiable, dangerous pathologies. Furthermore, it reinforces the conventional narrative of mental illness as a precursor to social violence as critiqued by Cassandra Kearney (2020). But I believe that the "flexible boundaries" in MHRR addressed by Molloy, Holladay, and Melonçon (2018, p. iv) must include the complex "rhetorical ecologies" (Edbauer, 2005) in which our work is situated, despite potential challenges to dominant approaches to our work.

Engagement in Two Voices

July 2020. Before leaving my childhood home for the last time, I look once more through the metal file cabinet in the den. Shoved to the back of the bottom drawer, I find a file folder labeled "Joe" in Dad's handwriting.

Inside are fragments of my parents' encounters with Joe, including a detailed log of run-ins with my brother used to secure orders of protection and a manila envelope containing letters he wrote. After Mom and Dad became too fearful to open the door when Joe stopped by, my brother began dropping off cards, letters, and an assortment of random items—his social security card, birth certificate, old photographs, and newspaper clippings—in their mailbox.

I wait months before reading what I've stumbled upon.

One feature of an interpretive autoethnographic methodology is the inclusion of "artifacts" that populate the ethnographic site (Denzin, 2014). In this section, I discuss two handwritten letters that Joe composed to suggest that notions of rhetoricity can be complicated in individuals displaying severe psychosis with anosognosia. One letter consists of 19 handwritten pages on yellowed legal paper written to our parents in 2015. The other, a three-page letter also composed on legal paper and addressed to me, was written in 2005 and mailed to my home address. Both letters constitute personal correspondence, making analysis of them potentially problematic from an ethical perspective. Writing about letters authored by an individual who is still living could be viewed as a violation of the letter writer's right to justify the rhetorical components evident in each document as well. I have attempted to mitigate these concerns somewhat by

- situating the letters in the "rhetorical ecology/ies" (Edbauer, 2005) within/ from which each was written
- limiting direct quotation, including only those words and phrases needed to support the argument
- acknowledging biases influencing the partiality of the analysis in the context of a methodological framework intended to focus on my interpretations of experiences with my sibling.

Analysis of the documents centers on two features important to demonstrating rhetoricity: first, agency in the form of positionality, or the features of his identity that Joe presents to his audience; and second, evidence of his openness to "affect*ability*" and "persuad*ability*," both criteria that Davis (2014) posited are conditions necessary for "symbolic interaction" (p. 2, emphasis in original).

November 2014. *In a moment of weakness, I fall for Joe's twisted logic and invite him to Birmingham for Thanksgiving. His current wife has left him, and he has nowhere to go.*

Joe makes it to town and calls me from a nearby gas station. He's slurring and growing agitated.

"I ca-ca-ca-can't find you. Y-Y-Y-You don't li-li-live where you sa-sa-said. I ne-ne-ne-need you to co-co-co-come g-g-get me," he stuttered into the phone.

After finally figuring out where Joe is, I climb into my car and head to the gas station. As soon as Joe steps foot outside the car, I know. There is something terribly, horribly, undeniably wrong with him.

Joe, my husband, and I spend four hours in the ER before the doctor decides Joe needs to stay overnight for further tests and observation. I send my husband home and spend the next ten hours slouched in a chair in my brother's hospital room, while Joe loudly mumbles incomprehensible utterances and engages in conversations with a host of invisible parties, screams for the floor nurse to bring him his knives (the four that were confiscated when Joe passed through the metal detector in the ER and set off the alarm), and swears at the doctor who informs us that Joe has suffered several TIAs, has exceedingly high blood pressure putting him at risk for stroke, tested positive for illicit drugs, and is likely reeling from the effects of taking himself off Lithium, a medication often prescribed for bipolar II disorder.

Eager to get us off the floor after my brother informs the doctor that he doesn't know what he's talking about and that we'll be going home, discharge orders are gathered: Take the medications prescribed, make an appointment immediately with your psychiatrist and GP, and stop carrying around knives. An attendant wheels Joe down to the first floor where my husband will pick us both up.

"I can't wait to eat Thanksgiving dinner, Sis," Joe said as he smiled up at me. "I told you there was nothing wrong with me."

"Ugh, just shut up," I replied, as we waited in silence for our ride.

"Dear Dad"

The letter addressed to both of our parents on the envelope but solely to our father in the salutation appeared in their mailbox a few months following the night I spent in the ER with my brother. By now, Joe is chronically homeless when he is not in jail or a rehab facility. He refuses to take prescribed medication and often gets booted from institutions where care is optional after pulling a knife on another resident or worker. Joe believes he has been wronged and that no one understands either how great he is or how badly he's suffered. Joe believes that much is owed to him, and his letter reflects this set of beliefs.

The letter's content is exceedingly redundant, as Joe engages in three problematic strategies that undercut efforts to demonstrate rhetoricity. The first is the inclusion of grandiose claims, some drawing on fragments of events that happened in the past but rewritten to support specific "rants" intended to be persuasive. For example, Joe provides excessive detail about tasks he undertook as a child growing up on the family farm, offering details such as the color and model of a specific grain wagon or the location of a field to a family he once knew. But the dates, estimates of bushels harvested, and potential market prices from 50 years ago are incongruous with the facts. Also, Joe greatly exaggerates his role in the farming operation, claiming that he, alone, "lined the pockets" of his family and is owed "millions of dollars in back pay, plus interest." At this particular point in Joe's life, he was desperate for money. The letter is just one of many efforts on his part to argue that he had not received the financial reward due to him from decades past. While not linked specifically to an argument regarding a potential mental illness, Joe's grandiose claims do reflect "confabulations" that Torrey (2012, p. 114) suggested are common among those suffering from severe psychosis and anosognosia.

Another feature of this letter is the appearance of (non)"recuperative ethos," a variation on "recuperative ethos" that Molloy (2020, pp. 122–124) submitted can be detected in individuals with mental illness who strive to assert credibility through "displays of astuteness" (pp. 125–127), "human connections" (pp. 127–131), and "religious topoi" (pp. 131–133). In his letter, Joe does rely on each category identified by Molloy in an attempt to re/gain ethos; however, the evidence offered consistently contradicts an ethical purpose. For instance, rather than asserting "experiential knowledge" as a sign of "astuteness" (p. 125), Joe brags about how many times he's been married and how many of his former wives have passed away—most through causes related to addiction. At one point in the letter, he poses a question to my father as the intended recipient: "Can you say you've been married that many times or lost that many exes? Well, I have." Or in demonstrating "human connections," Joe fills entire pages with the full names of individuals he knows, as well as the dates of birth and death for many. Included on these lists are also the names of celebrities Joe has never met personally, but claims as friends. These examples of (non)"-recuperative ethos" demonstrate largely failed attempts at rhetoricity, as Joe is unable to produce meaning that suggests an openness to "affect*ability*" or "persuad*ability*" as discussed by Davis (2014, p. 2, emphasis in original).

A final textual component of Joe's letter to our father is incorporation of "curses" in two senses. The first is in Joe's use of vulgar language, calling Dad everything from a "son of a b—" to a "c—-s—-r" to a "f—-g poor excuse for a man." And secondly, Joe conveys his hope that our father "dies a painful death," "loses everything he has," and a number of other horrific fates. Cursing is sprinkled throughout the letter indiscriminately. At points, Joe will follow the description of a fond memory with a sudden vulgar threat to kill Dad the next time he sees him. Perhaps most problematic is the closing of the letter, which Joe signs "Love, Your Son."

The document demonstrates a "richness" of the "rhetorical ecologies" (Edbauer, 2005) both driving and woven within the discursive space Joe occupies as the writer. At the same time, the illogical statements he presented throughout, perhaps representative of "agile epistemologies" that Molloy (2020) argued illustrate speakers' "engagement with language [that] might … [draw] on the rhetorical affordances that accompany their conditions" (p. 133), are too nonsensical to create a coherent argument. Simply put, rhetorical analysis is hindered by Joe's presentation of ideas, making it difficult to ascertain how Joe is eliciting specific ecological threads to convey his message.

"Dear Sister"

Joe's letter was mailed to me during what might be called a "honeymoon phase," recurrent in cycles of abuse during which abusers convey sorrow and regret and promise never to engage in abusive behavior again. Until they do. Several months before I received the letter, Joe and his fourth wife had visited me in Birmingham en route to Florida. At the time, I was undergoing treatment for a second bout of breast cancer; I laid stretched out on the couch across from my brother and his wife as we conversed, fighting off nausea from a recent round of chemo.

The tone of this document offers a stark contrast to the later letter written to my parents. Joe assumes a cordial relationship and adopts a sort of "aw, shucks, at least there's still time for me to get my life straightened out" persona. He couches this tone in the conventions of personal correspondence, opening the letter by mentioning that "it's Sunday morning" and the weather is rainy. Joe asks about my health and reveals that his high blood pressure has improved some since changing his diet, pretty "awesome," he says, for an "old man." Following a report on his health, Joe offers a snapshot of his wife's "bad back" and what her doctor said about possibly operating if the shots being administered don't do the trick.

Throughout the letter, Joe relies heavily on the language adopted by members of Alcoholics Anonymous (AA), specifically his attempts to "make things right" by trying to pay off some old personal "debts." He writes that "being a grandpa is a great joy," since "when [his] children were small [he] was a worthless drunk. A horrible man, and of course, brother." And while Joe adds "no excuses, it was my fault 100%," he focused much of the remainder of the letter on claims that he'd never done anything to hurt anyone. Joe ended the letter with an attempt to empathize with me, writing that despite the "awful time [he'd] had," referring to alcoholism, "you have been through much more misery than me with breast cancer." He says that he "sees that now." Following his closing, "I LOVE YOU, JOE," my sibling quotes a line from a Charlie Daniels' song, "It's a long road and a little wheel and it takes a lot of turns to get there," reinforcing the message that Joe's life journey has been progressive despite some bumps in the road.

Suggesting that Joe is perhaps insincere in his letter likely makes me sound cold and uncaring. Undoubtedly, the script of AA has helped many to atone for their actions and to rebuild their lives. At that particular moment in his life, Joe had discovered some momentary stability with his then-spouse who was also a recovering addict. Soon after mailing the letter, however, Joe spiraled out of control. He and his wife both resumed a lifestyle centered on drugs and alcohol, and Joe's violent, delusional behaviors took hold again. He had run-ins with the law for crimes including drug possession, illegal possession of weapons, and verbal and physical assault. Within three years, Joe was convicted of multiple counts of rape and spent time in a prison in Pennsylvania. While Joe had struggled with addiction since he was 13 years old, he attributed the "sins of [his] past," as he phrased it in the letter, solely to alcoholism. He hadn't entertained the possibility that severe mental illness had influenced him in a myriad of ways, including substance abuse. I provide details of this "ecological" context to explain why the rhetorical strategies presented in this document do not, from my partial perspective, constitute an openness to "persuad*ability*" or "affect*ability*" (Davis, 2014, p. 2).

Yes, But Also: Strategizing Interventional Spaces for Addressing Anosognosia in MHRR

As Cathryn Molloy and Lisa Melonçon (**this collection**) noted, "strategic interventions" can highlight "deliberate attempt[s] at change" and thus emphasize "intervention's ability to catalyze real and specific change and its propensity to break down silos in the process" (p. **2**). Drawing on the admittedly partial account I have presented in this chapter, I offer two specific interventions for MHRR.

Intervention #1: Expanding the Continuum to Address Severe Psychosis and Anosognosia

February 2013. Joe learns that one of his ex-wives and mother of two of his children has died. Reeling from the shock of losing a woman whom he'd beaten repeatedly, Joe showed up at our parents' house in a stupor.

My mom tearfully recounted the visit minutes after Joe left that evening, telling me through sobs that he "terrorized" her and my dad and threatened to push Dad, then 77 years old, down the basement stairs and "crack his head open on the concrete floor," since my brother claimed that "Dad never gave a damn about him or any of his wives."

After Mom convinced Joe to get out, my sibling proceeded to his daughter's house and threw her down a flight of stairs in front of her grade school-aged daughters. She sought medical attention in the ER for broken bones, bruises, and a concussion.

★★★★

Months later, Joe called me on my office phone, threatening to "come down to Alabama and kill your whole f——-g family if you don't send me some money." He'd been in jail for a few weeks and didn't have money for cigarettes.

"Why'd you change your home phone number, anyway? I've never done a damn thing to hurt any of you people," he screamed at me, forgetting, I guess, that he'd left vicious, threatening messages on our voice machine night after night until the tape ran out.

"Just because I was upset about losing the mother of my children," he continued, "you all think you can cut me out. Call me, B——-!"

Silence.

"Well, give me a call sometime, Sis. I'd love to see you," Joe quipped before he hung up.

As usual, conversations with Joe resembled recordings set to rewind. Threaten, accuse, excuse, reset.

Undoubtedly, rhetoric influences the ways in which human beings see, interpret, and name the phenomena that surround them. MHRR scholars should continue to prioritize humanist values in their work, encouraging both recognition and respect for individuals and populations who are often marginalized, ostracized, and silenced. **BUT**, MHRR needs to extend beyond a relatively safe continuum of mental health and illness constructions. As I have attempted to demonstrate, some who experience severe psychosis with anosognosia present real emotional and physical risks to themselves and others. And their potential lack of awareness of their disorders poses harm that it would be inhumane not to address through discursive and material actions.

Intervention #2: Expanding the Conversation to Give Voice to Cosurvivors

May 2021. I receive a phone call from Joe's case worker at the state hospital in Idaho. Joe has hightailed it out of Wyoming and is now seeking help elsewhere.

"He's signed a form so I can communicate with you about his care," she tells me. "I'm wondering if you could give me some information about his history."

We talk for over an hour. Mostly, it's me doing the talking and Joe's case worker writing it all down.

"I can tell you that your brother is really agitated," she offers after we've covered as much ground as either one of us can muster. "We have him in the maximum-security wing of the facility because he gets aggressive towards the staff when we say something he doesn't agree with. Also, we had to present a case to the 'Override Board' since Joe refused to take medication. He says there's nothing wrong with him and keeps trying to get the staff to call other hospitals in the area to get him released. We're pretty scared of him and what he might do."

"You should be," I responded.

A significant oversight in existing MHRR is the lived experience of mental illness from the perspective of cosurvivors, those individuals whose stories are **ALSO** imbricated in the rhetorical constructions and material ramifications of another's illness. The theoretical construct of "ambiguous loss," defined by Tehila Kovacs, Chaya Possick, and Eli Buchbinder (2018) as "longing" for a family member who may be physically present while not fulfilling the social role assigned to them (p. 1190), feels particularly fitting for the relationship I have shared with my brother. Rather than serving as a partner in crime, a protector, or a loving uncle to my daughters, Joe's presence (and threat) has factored into every aspect of my life. Rather than sharing decision-making regarding our parents' healthcare and final wishes as they aged, I strategize ways to keep them alive and respected by keeping Joe at bay. Instead of turning to my sibling for encouragement when I am unsure about choices I've made, I avoid listening to his cruel assessments of me and constantly doubt my strengths and my place in the world.

Ironically, the memories of Joe that I most struggle with are those that might be described as "good," the handful of moments I recall that make me smile. Joe's obsession with Don McLean's song "American Pie" and his insistence that he could find it playing any time, day or night, on the radio. His childlike response to learning various features on his first cell phone. These memories have led to existential crises for me that are largely rhetorical in nature. I question what I think I know about my brother and the identities that I have assigned to him in my quest to survive and to keep those I care for safe. I doubt what is "real" in our interactions. Joe's penchant for exploring his cell phone, for instance, soon became a means for terrorizing me and my family. My sibling's ability to turn his emotions on and off has had a profound effect on my interactions with others, as I question whether I can trust their intentions or believe what they tell me to be true. "Good" memories of Joe, in short, cause me to question everything, and these questions are tied to the rhetorical challenges seen in RHM and MHRR regarding what is "real" and what is "constructed" in our perceptions of bodies and minds.

Given the complexity suggested by scholars dabbling in MHRR, it is crucial that we recognize the vital role cosurvivors play in the "networked," "overlapping," "messy" "rhetorical ecologies" (Edbauer, 2005) that drive conversations about what it means to "be" mentally ill in contemporary society. J. Fred Reynolds (2018) noted that our shared history in RHM suggests that this field has become the "preferred home" for MHRR (p. 14). Amid the challenges posed by an attempt to devise meaning through snapshots of my lived experiences alongside my sibling, I have frequently reminded myself of Reynolds' assertion that these efforts constitute "work worth doing" (p. 14).

Acknowledgments

I want to thank Cathryn Molloy and Lisa Melonçon for their compassionate and rigorous guidance through numerous drafts of this chapter.

References

American Psychiatric Association. (2013). *Diagnostic and statistical manual of mental disorders.* (5th ed.). APA.

Berkenkotter, Carol. (2008). *Patient tales: Case histories and the uses of narrative in psychiatry.* University of South Carolina Press.

Davis, Diane. (2010). *Inessential solidarity: Rhetoric and foreigner relations.* University of Pittsburgh Press.

Denzin, Norman K. (2014). *Interpretive autoethnography.* (2nd ed.). University of Illinois Press.

Edbauer, Jenny. (2005). Unframing models of public distribution: From rhetorical situation to rhetorical ecologies. *Rhetoric Society Quarterly, 35*(4), 5–24.

Emmons, Kimberly. (2008). 'All on the list': Uptake in talk about depression. In Barbara Heifferon & Stuart C. Brown (Eds.), *Rhetoric of healthcare: Essays toward a new disciplinary inquiry* (pp. 159–180). Hampton Press.

Emmons, Kimberly. (2014). *Black dogs and blue words: Depression and gender in the age of self-care.* Rutgers University Press.

Foucault, Michel. (1965). *Madness and civilization: A history of insanity in the Age of Reason.* Trans. Alan Sheridan. Vintage Books.

Frances, Allen. (2013). *Saving normal: An insider's revolt against out-of-control psychiatric diagnosis, DSM-V, big pharma, and the medicalization of everyday life.* Harper Collins.

Goffman, Erving. (1961). *Asylum: Essays on the social situation of mental patients and other inmates.* Anchor Books.

Hanganu-Bresch, Cristina, & Berkenkotter, Carol. (2019). *Diagnosing madness: The discursive construction of the psychiatric patient, 1850–1920.* University of South Carolina Press.

Hinshaw, Stephen P. (2007). *The mark of shame: Stigma of mental illness and an agenda for change.* Oxford University Press.

Johnson, Jenell. (2010). The skeleton on the couch: The Eagleton affair, rhetorical disability, and the stigma of mental illness. *Rhetoric Society Quarterly, 40*(5), 459–478.

Kearney, Cassandra. (2020). A historical perspective on the 'mental illness as motive' narrative. *Rhetoric of Health and Medicine, 3*(1), 34–62.

Kovacs, Tehilia, Possick, Chaya, & Buchbinder, Eli. (2018). Experiencing the relationship with a sibling coping with mental health problems: Dilemmas of connection, communication, and role. *Health and Social Care in the Community, 27*, 1185–1192.

Lewiecki-Wilson, Cynthia. (2003). Rethinking rhetoric through mental disabilities. *Rhetoric Review, 22*(2), 156–167.

McCarthy, Lucille Parkinson. (1991). A psychiatrist using *DSM-III:* The influence of a charter document in psychiatry. In Charles Bazerman & James G. Paradis (Eds.), *Textual dynamics of the professions: Historical and contemporary studies of writing in professional communities* (pp. 358–378). University of Wisconsin Press.

Melonçon, Lisa, & Scott, J. Blake. (2018) Manifesting methodologies for the rhetoric of health and medicine. In L. Melonçon & J.B. Scott (Eds.), *Methodologies for the rhetoric of health and medicine* (pp. 1–23). Routledge.

Molloy, Cathryn. (2020). *Rhetorical ethos in health and medicine: Patient credibility, stigma, and misdiagnosis.* Routledge.

Molloy, Cathryn, Holladay, Drew, & Melonçon, Lisa. (2020). The place of mental health rhetoric research (MHRR) in *Rhetoric of Health and Medicine* and beyond. *Rhetoric of Health and Medicine, 3*(2), iii–x.

Porter, Roy. (2003). *Madness: A brief history.* Oxford University Press.

Prendergast, Catherine. (2001). On the rhetorics of mental disability. In James C. Wilson and Cynthia Lewiecki-Wilson (Eds.), *Embodied rhetorics: Disability in language and culture.* (pp. 45–60). Southern Illinois University Press.

Prendergast, Catherine. (2014). Mental disability and rhetoricity retold: The memoir on drugs. In David Bolt (Ed.), *Changing social attitudes toward disability: Perspectives from historical, cultural, and educational studies.* (pp. 60–67). Routledge.

Pryal, Katie Rose Guest. (2010). The genre of the mood memoir and the *ethos* of psychiatric disability. *Rhetoric Society Quarterly, 40*(5), 479–501.

Reynolds, J. Fred. (2018). A short history of mental health rhetoric research (MHRR). *Rhetoric of Health and Medicine, 1*(1–2), 1–18.

Reynolds, J. Fred, Mair, David C., & Fischer, Pamela C. (1992). *Writing and reading mental health records: Issues and analysis in professional writing and scientific rhetoric.* (1st ed.). Lawrence Erlbaum Associates, Inc.

Shorter, Edward. (1998). *A history of psychiatry: From the era of the asylum to the age of Prozac.* John Wiley & Sons, Inc.

Takayoshi, Pamela. (2020). Through the agency of words: Women in the American insane asylum, 1842-1890. *Rhetoric of Health and Medicine, 3*(2), 163–188.

Teston, Christa. (2017). *Bodies in flux: Scientific methods for negotiating medical uncertainty.* University of Chicago Press.

Torrey, E. Fuller. (2012). *The insanity offense: How America's failure to treat the seriously mentally ill endangers its citizens.* W.W. Norton and Co.

Uthappa, N. Renuka. (2017). Moving closer: Speakers with mental disabilities, deep disclosure, and agency through vulnerability. *Rhetoric Review, 36*(2), 164–175.

PART III

Pedagogical and Co-Curricular Interventions

10

TOWARD AN EMPATHY-FIRST APPROACH TO STUDENT MENTAL HEALTH

A Guide for Faculty Development

Lynn Reid

Introduction: Mental Health Misconceptions among College Instructors

Some years ago, during my work as a writing center tutor, I encountered a prompt for a literature course that asked students to "Demonstrate that the narrator of the 'Tell-Tale Heart' had a mental illness." The student I was working with was confident that their supporting evidence was exactly what the instructor was looking for: the narrator's use of repetition, his hallucinations, and his clear lack of remorse for the crime that had been committed, all topics that had been covered in class as part of a discussion about why the narrator was "crazy." It was clear to me that this assignment not only failed to define mental illness in any meaningful way, but it also very clearly "othered" anyone with a mental illness who may have been in that class. Mental illness, in this context, had been reduced to the "crazy" characteristics of a literary villain rather than addressed with the empathy the topic so deeply deserves. While the prompt above is, of course, quite problematic itself, it is reflective of a much broader concern: a lack of awareness on the part of many faculty regarding the realities of mental health and mental disability that significant numbers of students experience. This chapter intervenes in this lack of awareness by sharing details on a workshop I designed to help faculty to better appreciate students' mental health concerns and to respond to such struggles with empathy first.

The fact that college students need mental health support is well documented. National studies of college staff find that more than 90% of respondents report spending a significant amount of their working time focused on mental health concerns (Jashick, 2020)—percentages that have increased dramatically over the past decade (Eisenberg, 2019). A number of studies report

DOI: 10.4324/9781003144854-14

that postsecondary faculty—the employees that students are likely to interact with the most—are inadequately prepared to support students who may be struggling with their mental health. In a survey of 168 faculty members, for example, Karin Brockelman and Anna Scheyett (2015) found that "faculty may not be recognizing warning signs and symptoms of mental illness in students, making it difficult for them to provide students with support and assistance" (p. 347). These results align with a study of faculty awareness of students with disabilities, which indicated that "students with learning or mental health disabilities may encounter significantly more attitudinal barriers than those with physical disabilities" (Sniatecki, Perry, & Snell, 2015, p. 266).

A lack of awareness about these topics can have dire consequences for students. Those students who struggle to focus, fail to complete work, and otherwise disengage from a course can easily be written off as "not college material," yet these and many other indicators of poor performance can also be clear signs that a student is in distress and would benefit more from a supportive environment than from consistent reminders that they are underperforming. In "Are You Being Rigorous or Just Intolerant: How to Promote Mental Health in the College Classroom," Catherine Savini (2016) described her own experience learning to move beyond assuming that "bad" student behaviors were indicative of disengagement and instead shifted to a more empathetic approach that would allow increased flexibility to accommodate her students' often invisible needs. Of particular interest is Savini's focus on conceptions of "rigor" as a barrier to inclusive teaching. She explained,

> I always took pride in being 'a hard teacher.' I was rigorous but fair; my students didn't need to be geniuses to succeed, they just needed to be 'good students.' A good student attends class, sits attentively, participates in discussions, and meets deadlines.
>
> *(par. 1)*

Importantly, too often, student behaviors that may indicate a need for support are conflated with the behaviors of "bad students."

The notion that "good students" are those who follow the rules for behavior and timeliness in class is rooted in a broader discourse of rigor and grit that permeates academia. The *Chronicle of Higher Education* is often rife with such examples, including Scott Hippensteel's (2013) piece "Be Hard to Get Along With," which argued for the need for faculty to emphasize respect and decorum in their classrooms. Hippensteel included examples that range from students who leave class for a 30-minute lunch and then come back and demand that their questions be answered to those who ask for extensions or makeup exams. While there is an obvious problem with a student strolling out of class simply to take a lunch break, that Hippensteel placed that in the same category of behavior as a student missing an exam or asking that an answer to a question in class be repeated is troubling and reflects ableist assumptions that students can all perform equally if they simply choose to be present, pay attention, or manage their time effectively. As David Webster and Nicola Rivers (2019) noted,

> the turn towards an uncritical narrative of 'they need to be more resilient/tougher/less soft' does [students] no favours. In fact, at worst, such narratives of resilience can feed into toxic cultural discourses that position current generations of young people as 'snowflakes' who are easily 'triggered'.
>
> *(p. 2)*

These pervasive discourses can (and, indeed, often do) serve to silence students whose behaviors do not clearly align with assumptions about acceptable student behavior in postsecondary settings.

Yet, demanding that students demonstrate resilience and grit does little to support students who are struggling with mental health. In fact, some of the same behaviors that are often cited as markers of a "bad" student can be misleading, as "academic failure, course repetition, and academic attrition were common results of mental health problems" (Markoulakis & Kirsh, 2013, p. 92). For students who are struggling with mental health, these poor performance outcomes can be aligned with symptomatic behavior, including avoiding situations and social events that require participation, difficulty adhering to strict due dates, low energy levels, difficulty coping with stressors, and poor attendance (Markoulakis & Kirsh, 2013). Unfortunately, however, faculty can easily assume that such behaviors are markers of lazy students rather than of a deeper underlying concern. Karin Brockelman and Anna Scheyett (2015) found that

> Despite the high rates of mental health issues among university students (estimated 15% of students), [a] survey of university faculty revealed the surprising fact that common symptoms of mental illnesses were not noted even once per year by a substantial proportion of respondents (e.g., about 50% did not see withdrawal, a common symptom of depression, even once a year). Faculty may not be recognizing warning signs and symptoms of mental illness in students, making it difficult for them to provide students with support and assistance.
>
> *(pp. 346–347)*

That faculty may conflate potential symptoms of a mental health crisis with disengagement or an inability to meet the demands of collegiate expectations is problematic, and their responses to such scenarios may further contribute to negative self-perception and stigma regarding mental health on the part of students (Rickerson et al., 2004). With these issues and problems in mind, I designed a workshop for faculty meant to offer them crucial information on student mental health. Below, I share details on that workshop such that readers interested in developing similar workshops at their own institutions might adapt my framework for helping faculty and staff to show empathy first when faced with behaviors that could be signs of mental distress.

Introduction to Faculty Development Workshop

In an effort to help faculty better support students who may be struggling with mental health on my own campus, I designed a faculty development workshop with the goals of raising awareness of how mental health might impact classroom behavior and encouraging instructors to engage their students with an eye toward empathy rather than rigidly defined (and, at times, inherently ableist) expectations for behavior and performance. Often, well-intentioned instructors argue that they would be more than happy to extend flexibility to students who openly communicate their struggles to the professor (a topic that I return to in more depth below). This workshop was intended to help faculty to realize that perhaps more than they realize, students are communicating their struggles through the behaviors that they exhibit in the classroom. The problem, however, is that this communication is obscured by a dominant metanarrative that aligns student success with grit and rigor, and thus, instructors with the best of intentions often believe that they are supporting students' needs by enforcing strict policies surrounding attendance, deadlines, and classroom behavior. In reality, their assumptions about these behaviors may be rooted in ableist expectations that can obscure the mental health needs of many students.

To address these concerns, I designed my workshop with two central aims: (1) To help faculty develop a more complex understanding of student behaviors and (2) To encourage faculty to demonstrate empathy to students who are unable to exhibit the behaviors of a "good" student, regardless of whether students disclose a specific mental health struggle.

Workshop Materials and Rationale

The primary resources for this workshop are narrative-based materials, including sample student scenarios for discussion and excerpts of student narratives from *The Mighty*—a crowdsourced publication that promotes first-person accounts from people living with disabilities, including those related to mental health. My choice to work with narrative as the primary method of persuasion is rooted in narrative medicine, where narrative-based training is utilized as a means of fostering empathy for patients and shifting to a patient-centered ethic of care (Marini, 2018); narrative medicine relies on the cultivation of empathy through storytelling (Blakenship, 2019; Nussbaum, 1998). By focusing on students' stories, I hoped that faculty would begin to see opportunities for empathy where they may have previously observed a need for grit and rigor.

As Amy Vidali (2015) suggested, it is important to "[bring] the insights of disabled people and perspectives in order to innovate, include, and transgress expected and exclusionary norms" (p. 33). By emphasizing narratives in the workshop, I hoped to illustrate both the realities of some students' lived experiences and opportunities for faculty to reconsider ableist course policies that do not accommodate mental health needs.

Table Discussions of Sample Scenarios

At the start of the workshop, I distributed index cards that each contained one sample scenario drawn from the list below.

- A student has a habit of getting up and walking out of class.
- A student consistently misses class when there are quizzes or exams scheduled.
- A student consistently comes to class without handing in any writing.
- A student's behavior is consistently disruptive to class.
- A student suddenly begins to accrue a lot of absences.
- A student falls asleep in class regularly.
- A student always seems distracted in class; you hear a rumor that they spend a lot of time "partying."

Faculty then worked in small groups for about 15 minutes to brainstorm answers to two questions based on the reading of their scenario:

1 How would you respond to this student?
2 What assumptions about the reasons for their behavior influence your response?

Group Discussion of Sample Scenarios

Following the small group activity, I brought participants back to the larger group to review their responses to the various student scenarios and the assumptions that informed their responses.

Some common responses from faculty included:

- A student who consistently misses class when there are quizzes or exams scheduled is avoiding the tests because they haven't studied.
- A student who consistently comes to class without handing in any writing needs to work on their time management.
- A student whose behavior is consistently disruptive to class is challenging the instructor's authority.

- A student who suddenly begins to accrue a lot of absences isn't taking the class seriously.

These common responses are revealing in terms of what faculty often assume is motivating the behaviors that are deemed undesirable for college students. The dominant narratives that suggest that students are "academically adrift" (Arum, 2011) and lacking in grit and should, therefore, not be "coddled" by faculty are reproduced in the name of preparing students for the "real" world and, I would argue, often come from a place of good intentions. Many faculty truly believe that they are doing students a disservice with policies and expectations that are too flexible or that appear to enable students to take the path of least resistance. The question, then, is how to encourage faculty to move toward a more empathetic approach to student behavior that acknowledges the myriad ways that mental health can impact a student's ability to, in Margaret Price's (2011) terms, "pass" as neurotypical and nondisabled (p. 7) and thereby perform the role of a "good" student.

Providing an Alternate Reading

To challenge these assumptions about grit and rigor, I provided a more detailed description of what might be happening from a students' point of view for each scenario. These descriptions were all taken from my own experiences with students (with identifying information modified to protect privacy) and serve as an intervention intended to challenge the master narrative that those students who complete their work on time, attend class regularly, and persist through obstacles by relying on grit are "good" students, while those who may struggle to focus, miss class frequently, and are unable to overcome obstacles are "bad" students. Below, I share the original scenarios with the fuller stories that I used in the workshop.

Scenario 1

- A student has a habit of getting up and walking out of class when group work is assigned.

Kevin got up and left class for an average of 10 or 15 minutes during most class periods during the semester, essentially missing all the group work for the course. When I informed him that this behavior would have a negative impact on his grade because he was missing so much class time, Kevin told me that he has severe social anxiety and would time his departures to stave off panic attacks and that the loss of points was an acceptable cost to pay to preserve his mental health.

Scenario 2

• A student consistently comes to class without handing in any writing.

Malik came to every class, but never had any work to hand in. He would try to spend class time working on the assignment that was due that day, but often wasn't able to finish and ultimately failed the class. At the end of the semester, knowing that he had already failed, Makik came to my office hours to tell me that he had just been diagnosed with major depression.

> I didn't know what was happening. It was like I was frozen, and I couldn't get out of bed in the morning. And then I couldn't concentrate on my schoolwork or complete any assignments that required a lot of thinking.

Scenario 3

• A student always seems distracted in class and you hear a rumor that they spend a lot of time partying.

Toni couldn't sit still in class and often appeared to derail class discussions by introducing a new tangent that was unrelated to the topic at hand. Her grades began to slip, and she seemed to no longer care about her performance in the class. One day when Toni was absent, another classmate loudly informed everyone that Toni was probably hungover from all the drinking she did at a party the night before—something that had become a regular occurrence. A few weeks later, Toni came to my office to inform me that she might seem even more distracted than usual in class because she was just prescribed medication for bipolar disorder. This was a new diagnosis and, although her mom had bi-polar, Toni was shocked and embarrassed to now be in the same boat. "I was self-medicating," Toni said. "I drank and got all of these new piercings because I thought it would make me feel better, but my mind just kept racing."

Unpacking the Scenarios

Certainly, these examples do not suggest that the students described are "bad" students—they are each obviously struggling with their mental health and would benefit from empathy more than an approach that emphasizes rigor and grit. Instructors in these workshops overwhelmingly expressed empathy in response to the stories above, even though mental health had been the furthest thing from most of their minds during their initial discussion of the sample scenarios. Thus, presenting the backstory to each scenario helped instructors to consider that perhaps those behaviors students' behaviors could be signs of mental health struggles warranting empathy rather than signs of apathy or disengagement.

Presentation of Excerpts from "The Mighty"

I was pleased that using the short scenarios were largely effective as they did elicit empathy in workshop participants through shedding additional light onto situations that were easy to mistake for student apathy or absence of rigor. Once instructors were primed to interpret student behavior from a position of empathy through the scenarios, the next questions focused on how an instructor might best respond to a student who is demonstrating what they deem as problematic behavior. As noted above, time is one of the most significant barriers to students who are struggling with mental health, specifically in terms of expected time in the classroom and submission of assignments. Fortunately for faculty who strive to create inclusive spaces for students who struggle with mental health, the ways that time is allocated and extended in a course are largely left to their discretion. Yet, as Frederic Fovet (2020) noted, little attention has been explicitly paid to how principles of universal design might also inform class policies and expectations for behavior regarding mental health conditions in postsecondary settings. An approach that adheres to principles of universal design is one that "maximizes the usability of educational materials and environments for all students by anticipating a variety of student needs," thereby "minimiz[ing] the need for special accommodations" (Rickerson et al., 2004). Fovet's study provided important insights into some of the specific classroom policies that can impede the success of students who are struggling with mental health, including: deadlines, participation grades, and expectations for social interactions. To approach these and other concerns from a universal design perspective requires faculty to recognize mental health's impact on the ways that students engage with a course rather than simply assuming that a student who fails to meet a standard of "college-level behavior" simply does not care about their performance in the course.

To facilitate a translation of empathy for student experiences elicited by narratives about mental health into concrete adaptations to teaching in faculty development, it is useful for faculty to understand the concept of "crip time" (Samuels, 2017; Wood, 2017). "Crip time" is a term commonly used to denote the ways that normative conceptions of time and punctuality may fail to accommodate the needs of people with disabilities, including mental health conditions. In short, "Crip time challenges ableist normativity and recognizes diverse bodies and minds by redefining time" (Ljuslinder et al., 2020, p. 36) in ways that account for individual needs.

To illustrate how an understanding of "crip time" might influence faculty expectations about student behavior, I turned to narrative excerpts from *The*

Mighty that focus on student attendance in the context of mental health. Selections from *The Mighty* that focus on the experiences of students who struggle with mental health reinforce a counternarrative to the dominant discourses that position underperforming students as lacking discipline or motivation.

Among the many topics related to mental health and student behavior in the selections I used, the narratives that address class attendance are perhaps the most eye-opening to instructors who are just beginning to learn about the countless ways that mental health might impact the way a student engages with a course and the disproportionate impact of ableist policies on students who struggle with mental health. (See Appendix for links to these and additional related articles that could be used in similar workshops.)

To frame this discussion at the workshop, I shared excerpts from the following pieces:

- "Stop Lying to Your Professors About Your Depression (And Other Ways I Learned to Survive College)" by Maria Giacchino
- "To the Professor Who Dismissed My Bipolar Disorder" by Christina McCullough
- "Dear Professor, Here's the Real Reason I Missed Your Class Again" by Alizabeth Stachlinski
- "What I Wish My College Community Advisors Had Known About Me" by Sarah Oling

These examples all directly address the ways that strict policies regarding attendance in class can be detrimental to students who are struggling with mental health, which I demonstrated by pulling out some select quotes to share with faculty in the workshop. In one example, Maria Giacchino (2016) wrote about her experience seeking accommodations (as required by her university) for depression, revealing that while a letter of accommodation was sufficient for extra time on tests and quizzes, she had no official documentation to address the ways that her depression might impact attendance. She explained, "So, my second attempt to avoid telling my professors I had depression was to lie, like many college students do to avoid coming to class or facing a deadline" (par. 9), followed by some sample emails that include some of the ways she attempted to address her needs by describing fake problems to her professor.

Writing about her experience with bipolar disorder as a college student, Christina McCullough (2018) addressed her piece in *The Mighty* "To the Professor Who Dismissed My Bipolar Disorder." McCullough's narrative reflected on her journey and how she "fought and clawed [her] way through" years of struggle with her mental health, including failing out of college when she was first diagnosed at 18. As a returning adult student more than two decades later, McCullough wrote about asking a professor for an extension to make up an exam as she regained her ability to focus after a period of crisis, to which the professor replied, "I don't do that. I've never heard of anyone doing that." To further illustrate her experience, McCullough wrote:

> Two and a half weeks ago, I started to teach myself the content from your course. I worked very hard on it. I hired a tutor, who I paid for myself. I started to feel confident with the material. I just needed a bit more time. Just a week would have given me a total of three and a half weeks to learn an entire term's worth of material. But I knew I could do it. After such a long time in such a self-loathing and dark place, when I feel confident about something so early after coming out of it, it's genuine. I was even enjoying the content.
>
> That was my mindset when I met with you today. I came to you, binder in hand, ready to show you my work, my progress and my dedication to doing well in your course. But you dismissed me, questioned why I even took the course, if I didn't "need" it, and told me that there was nothing you could do. I needed to talk to someone else. I was a mere irritation that you didn't have time for.
>
> *(Par. 9)*

As the narratives above from *The Mighty* make clear, rigid attendance policies can also be harmful to students who are struggling with mental health, as bad days cannot readily be predicted in advance. Such policies are, as many scholars and disability activists have noted, ableist in their demands that all bodies and minds adhere to a normative schedule that prioritizes accountability over students' individual needs. The workshop addresses this issue by sharing these narratives in which students' complex mental health struggles account for their need for more flexibility. However, another issue the workshop needed to address was the complications with disclosure in the context of stigma.

"If They Would Just Tell Me": Stigma and the Politics of Disclosure

Instructors in the workshop were quick to point out that they'd be more than happy to extend empathy and flexibility when a student makes them aware of a specific issue, particularly one that is related to mental health. Karin Brokelman and Anna Scheyett's (2015) survey similarly found that, in instances when faculty were aware of students' mental health concerns, they were frequently willing to provide accommodations such as extended deadlines and to connect students to counseling and other support services on campus. While this is a step in the right direction, instructors may not realize what a big ask it is for students to reveal such personal information, particularly considering the stigma that frequently surrounds mental health and the fear that a diagnosis might be conflated with one's entire identity (Green et al., 2020; Kerschbaum, 2014). To acknowledge the student perspective, the workshop includes a discussion of scholarship in the field of Mental Health Rhetoric Research (MHRR), which reveals that decisions about disclosure are often mediated by institutional politics and policies that can pose tangible risks for a person who discloses a mental health diagnosis. In many accounts, MHRR researchers recount their own experiences seeking accommodations—experiences that are often described as painful, uncomfortable, or even blatantly discriminatory. Ann Green et al. (2020) outlined the many ways that requests for accommodations can be misread in a manner similar to the student scenarios presented above: "Asking for a later teaching time, for example, can be viewed as 'lazy' rather than a reasonable accommodation for the effects of a new medication" (p. 12). Others write about avoiding disclosure altogether to avoid experiencing negative stigma (Vidali, 2015) in an attempt to "pass" as neurotypical (Kafer, 2016). While faculty may see themselves as empathetic and flexible to students who share their challenges, the workshop uses these texts to emphasize that students may not have had positive experiences with disclosure in the past and/or might not trust that their instructors will not reinforce problematic stigmas about mental health. Thus, the discussion leads to the call for instructors to avoid eliciting disclosures.

At the same time, most professors have worked with students who supply excuses rather than produce the assigned work, and I would be remiss to not admit that students occasionaly lie about the circumstances that prevent them from attending class or taking exams. Shifting the discussion back to Giacchino's story from *The Mighty*, however, reveals that some of these lies may be hiding a truth that a student is afraid or embarrassed to reveal. For Giacchino, lies about computer problems and other obstacles that caused her to "accidentally" miss material from class are more comfortable than facing potential stigma about her mental health from a professor.

The workshop also included a discussion of Melissa Nicolas (2017), who recommended that attendance policies be constructed to allow flexibility between instructors and students to negotiate their needs together. This move provides students with some needed agency in determining the course of their progress (Wood, 2017). Likewise, rather than emphasize situations that will be considered "exceptions" to a mandated policy, Tara Wood (2017) suggested that all scenarios be open for discussion. Bringing these texts into the workshop serve as examples to illustrate both why and how faculty might move away from a medical model of disability that grants exceptions based on diagnoses and documentation, toward a social model that redesigns policies and spaces for inclusivity.

Workshop Feedback

I have offered this workshop in a one- to two-hour format a total of four times for a range of audiences, including an interdisciplinary group of faculty on my campus, full and part-time instructors in my writing program (with a representative from our university's counseling center), and colleagues at regional and national conferences. Overwhelmingly, the feedback I have received during follow-up discussions with attendees has been positive, particularly among instructors who teach developmental-level courses and among representatives from our university counseling center.

Despite this enthusiasm, though, I did get some pushback—particularly on the notion that instructors should extend empathy to students by providing more flexible opportunities for participation and engagement as it relates to issues of faculty labor. Faculty—and particularly those who work on part-time and contingent contracts—argue that policies that prohibit late assignments or make-up exams and that demand student attendance and active engagement during class are necessary so that they can manage their own workloads. This is certainly a valid concern, and as I note in the workshop, having structures in place can also be helpful even to students who struggle to meet expectations. In response to such critiques, I suggest that faculty simply consider how they respond to those students who are failing to adhere to standards of "good" student behavior. For example, when a student falls behind on coursework or is consistently submitting things late, acknowledging that it can be hard to keep up when things are stressful and reminding students that, in addition to tutoring support, the campus also offers counseling, might be more appropriate than simply issuing a zero and telling the student to get organized. Similarly, if a student begins to accumulate absences and is often late to class, welcoming them when they are present rather than shaming them with something like, "Well I'm glad you've decided to join us today" might communicate to a student who is struggling that they are in a safe space. Even in instances when students are unable to complete the requirements of a course and earn an F, I remind faculty that they can tell students that sometimes other things get in the way of school, and that it's important to take time to think about the extent to which obstacles were within the students' ability to control and what resources might be available for the next time around. In short, extending empathy doesn't have to mean eliminating all requirements; it simply means that faculty should be cautious not to assume that a student is performing poorly because they are lazy, disorganized, or apathetic. Such assumptions can lead to inappropriate responses to students that could even exacerbate the mental health concerns that could be the root of their behaviors to begin with. Responding with empathy first allows for the possibility that the student's performance is the result of a mental health struggle rather than the result of a character flaw, a sign of laziness, or an indication of apathy. With that, we also discuss the limitations of disclosure, as not every student who is struggling may have a diagnosis and not all students who are struggling necessarily are doing so because of their mental health. I argue, however, that an empathy-first approach benefits *all* students, regardless of diagnosis or factors beyond mental health that may impact their behavior in class. Using empathy as a lens and mental health as an example helps instructors to reframe their responses to student behavior across a range of scenarios, all of which can benefit students who choose not to disclose the details of their personal circumstances.

Advice for Those Interested in Adapting this Workshop

One important consideration for adapting this workshop for any local context is faculty buy-in. As is often the case when discussing issues related to structural inequalities in higher education, participants in the workshop may express resistance to a suggestion that their established practices may cause harm to a population of students. In my experience, I have found that using narratives to reframe faculty perceptions of student behavior throughout the course of the workshop—several times if needed—has quelled some of this resistance.

Additionally, it is also important to remind faculty that they are not in a position to diagnose or treat students who may exhibit symptoms of a mental health disability. It can be helpful to have a member of the counseling staff available to answer any faculty questions regarding their role in supporting students' mental health and to have resources for local mental health support ready to share. Likewise, while the workshop is intended to raise faculty awareness about student mental health, the ultimate goal is to foster compassion and empathy for all students who may be exhibiting behaviors that a faculty member may interpret as a lack of motivation or engagement. I have found that it is often necessary to recenter that goal throughout the course of the workshop.

Finally, like any other professional development subject, this topic should be revisited regularly in future conversations so that faculty can contribute their own experiences and evolving perceptions of student behavior and mental health. Frequent reminders of how a student's struggles with mental health may manifest in the classroom along with strategies for academically supporting such students are necessary for the impact of the workshop to solidify.

Conclusion

Though narratives about student mental health serve as a first step to help faculty members to identify normative classroom practices that can have an exclusionary effect or, as Frederic Fovet (2020) suggested, could even further exacerbate a students' mental health conditions, adopting an ethic of care is not accomplished through storytelling alone. To effectively train faculty to adopt a more flexible approach to their interactions with students who may be struggling with mental health, it is necessary to shift the paradigm of discussion from accountability to access. Faculty must be mindful of the fact that interactions with students are complicated by power dynamics and privacy concerns, which means that students may be unwilling to disclose the specifics of their struggles. The approaches I have suggested in the discussion-based workshop I describe above for opening a dialogue about student mental health do not constitute a panacea. Despite this fact, the above recommendations for faculty development and classroom practice do introduce a counternarrative to the notion that students who struggle with some of the behaviors that are expected at the postsecondary level are simply lazy or disengaged. Changing the dominant narrative about student performance is, I believe, an essential step toward creating a more inclusive environment for the many students for whom mental health is an occasional or persistent barrier to perceived success in college. Positive steps toward this goal have been taken as a result of the COVID-19 pandemic as faculty have, for example, adopted flexible policies (Stommel, 2020), encouraged multiple methods of class participation, and relaxed attendance requirements; the challenge for faculty development is to sustain this momentum as higher education shifts to the "new normal" that is on the horizon.

References

Arum, Richard, & Roska, Josipa. (2011). *Academically adrift: Limited learning on college campuses.* The University of Chicago Press.

Blakenship, Lisa. (2019). *Changing the subject: A theory of rhetorical empathy.* Utah State University Press.

Brockelman, Karin F., & Scheyett, Anna M. (2015). Faculty perceptions of accommodations, strategies, and psychiatric advance directives for university students with mental illnesses. *Psychiatric Rehabilitation Journal, 38*(4), 342–348. https://doi.org/10.1037/prj0000143

Eisenberg, Daniel. (2019). Countering the troubling increase in mental health symptoms among U.S. college students. *Journal of Adolescent Health, 65*(5), 573–574.

Fovet, Frederic. (2020, March 1). *Exploring the potential of universal design for learning with regards to mental health issues in higher education* [Paper presentation]. Pacific Rim International Conference on Disability and Diversity Conference Proceedings. Honolulu, Hawai'i. https://scholarspace.manoa.hawaii.edu/bitstream/10125/69333/Exploring_the_Potential_of_Universal_Design_for_Learning_with_Regards_to_Mental_Health_Issues_in_Higher_Education_Fovet.pdf.

Giacchino, Maria. (2016, Sept 10). Stop lying to professors about your depression (and other ways I learned to survive college). *The Mighty.* https://themighty.com/2016/09/how-to-tell-college-professors-about-your-depression/

Green, Ann, Alyssa, Dura, Lucia, Harris, Patrick, Heilig, Leah, Kirby, Bailey, McClintick, Jay, Pfender, Emily, & Carrasco, Rebecca. (2020). Teaching and researching with a mental health diagnosis: Practices and perspectives on academic ableism. *Rhetoric of Health & Medicine, 3*(2). http://medicalrhetoric.com/journal/3-2/green/

Hippensteel, Scott. (2013, Oct 23). Be hard to get along with. *The Chronicle of Higher Education.* https://www.chronicle.com/article/be-hard-to-get-along-with/

Jashick, Scott. (2020, Mar 26). Student affairs leaders on mental health, race relations, free speech, and more. *Inside Higher Ed.* https://www.insidehighered.com/news/survey/student-affairs-leaders-mental-health-race-relations-free-speech-and-more

Kafer, Alison. (2016). Un/safe disclosures: Scenes of disability and trauma. *Journal of Literary & Cultural Disability Studies, 10*(1), 1–20. https://www.muse.jhu.edu/article/611309

Kerschbaum, Stephanie. (2014). On rhetorical agency and disclosing disability in academic writing. *Rhetoric Review, 33*(1), 55–71.
https://compositionforum.com/issue/32/anecdotal-relations.php

Ljuslinder, Karin, Ellis, Katie, & Vikström, Lotta. (2020) Cripping time: Understanding the life course through the lens of ableism. *Scandinavian Journal of Disability Research, 22*(1): 35–38 https://doi.org/10.16993/sjdr.710

Marini M.G. (2019) Between Narrative Medicine and Storytelling in the Healthcare Ecosystem: Narrative Medicine and Medical Humanities and Their Impact on Education and Training of Healthcare Providers. In: *Languages of Care in Narrative Medicine.* Springer, Cham. https://doi.org/10.1007/978-3-319-94727-3_4

Markoulakis, Roula, & Kirsh, Bonnie. (2013). Difficulties for university students with mental health problems: A critical interpretive synthesis. *Review of Higher Education, 37*(1), 77–100.

McCullough, Christine. (2018, Dec 15) To the professor who dismissed my bipolar disorder. *The Mighty.* https://themighty.com/2018/12/letter-to-professor-about-bipolar/

Nicolas, Melissa. (2017). Ma(r)king difference: Challenging ableist assumptions in writing program policies. *WPA: Writing Program Administration, 40*(3), 10–22.

Nussbaum, Martha C. (1998). *Cultivating humanity. A classical defense of reform in liberal education.* Harvard University Press.

Oling, Sarah. (2017, Apr 21). What I wish my college community advisors had known about me. *The Mighty. https://themighty.com/u/sarah-oling/*

Price, Margaret. (2014). *Mad at School: Rhetorics of mental disability and academic life.* The University of Michigan Press.

Rickerson, Nancy, Souma, Alfred, & Burgstahler, Sheryl. (2004, March 31–April 1). *Psychiatric disabilities in postsecondary education: Universal design, accommodations and supported education* [Paper presentation]. National Capacity Building Institute Issues of Transition and Postsecondary Participation for Individuals with Hidden Disabilities, Honolulu, Hawai'i. http://www.ncset.hawaii.edu/institutes/mar2004/papers/pdf/Souma_revised.pdf.

Samuels, Ellen. (2017). Six ways of looking at crip time. *Disability Studies Quarterly, 37*(3). https://dsq-sds.org/article/view/5824/4684

Savini, Catherin. (2016, May 4). Are we being rigorous or just intolerant? How to promote mental health in the college classroom. *The Chronicle of Higher Education.* https://www.chronicle.com/article/Are-You-Being-Rigorous-or-Just/236341

Sniatecki, Jessica, Perry, Holly, & Snell, Linda. (2015). Faculty attitudes and knowledge regarding college students with disabilities. *Journal of Postsecondary Education and Disability, 28*(3), 259–275.

Stachlinski, Alizabeth. (2017, Mar 7). Dear professor, here's the real reason I missed your class again. *The Mighty.* https://themighty.com/2017/03/what-to-tell-professor-class-anxiety/

Stommel, Jesse. (2020). Designing for care: Hybrid pedagogy in the time of COVID-19. *The Blue Dot,* 12. https://d1c337161ud3pr.cloudfront.net/files%2Fd0682ab5-7f94-492d-ab68-b7110a3b6764_The%20Blue%20DOT-Issue%2012.pdf

Vidali, Amy. (2015). Disabling writing program administration. *WPA: Writing Program Administration, 38*(2), 32–55.

Wood, Tara. (2017). Cripping time in the college composition classroom. *College Composition and Communication, 69*(2), 260–282.

Webster, David R., & Rivers, Nicola. (2018). Resisting resilience: Disrupting discourses of self-efficacy. *Pedagogy Culture and Society, 27*(4), 523–535.

APPENDIX

https://themighty.com/2016/09/how-to-tell-college-professors-about-your-depression/

https://themighty.com/2018/12/letter-to-professor-about-bipolar/

https://themighty.com/2017/04/depression-college-community-advisors/

https://themighty.com/2017/03/what-to-tell-professor-class-anxiety/

https://themighty.com/2017/06/professor-medication-bipolar-disorder-advice/

https://themighty.com/2018/08/counseling-professor-got-wrong-about-bipolar-disorder-mania/

https://themighty.com/2016/08/letter-to-professor-who-needs-a-better-understanding-of-mental-illness/

https://themighty.com/2016/06/letter-to-the-teacher-who-used-ocd-as-an-adjective/

https://themighty.com/2017/03/letter-to-teacher-about-struggles-anxiety/

https://themighty.com/2017/12/participation-points-college-class-anxiety-mental-health/

https://themighty.com/2020/01/attendance-policies-hurt-disabled-students/

11

"DO YOU FEEL LIKE ☹": DISCURSIVE INTERVENTIONS IN UNIVERSITY MENTAL HEALTH RHETORICS

Leslie R. Anglesey and Adam Hubrig

Introduction

University mental health centers across the United States describe themselves as "committed to promoting well-being" (University of Chicago, n.d.), able to "improve academic performance" (Georgetown University, n.d.) and interested in students' well-being, as in one university health center web banner that directs students to a login portal and asks: "do you feel like :(?" (Clemson, n.d.). Through these articulations, the very concept of mental health is rhetorically constructed alongside the role of institutions of higher education in mental health concerns. Drawing on textual analysis through qualitative coding of university websites, our chapter intervenes in the rhetorical project through which counseling centers—acting as an extension of their larger institutional homes—frame universities as proactive intercessors in the mental health and well-being of students. Our findings from this project highlight a troubling trend in these websites' presentations of mental health services as marketed by campuses—they foreground academic productivity as the goal of mental health services. Furthermore, we argue many of these articulations of mental health *as a means to* academic success pathologize mental health concerns, ultimately blaming students for the ableist structures of institutions of higher education. Our analysis seeks to intervene in these unmediated representations of mental health by examining the rhetorical construction of mental health on universities' institutionally sanctioned websites.

To understand the rhetorical construction of mental health on campus, this chapter draws on mental health rhetoric methodologies rooted in textual analysis (Reynolds, Mair, & Fischer, 2013; Yergeau & Huebner, 2017). In reviewing how US universities construct mental health rhetorics through their own

DOI: 10.4324/9781003144854-15

presentation of mental health services on campus, we found these institutions frequently framed themselves as benevolent arbiters of "mental health" while distancing themselves from being sites of trauma and places where students can be pathologized. Drawing from a pool of 39 US university websites, we gathered a corpus of public-facing resources as they pertain to mental health services. Combining textual analysis with qualitative coding, we explored how universities construct mental health within their institutions. By applying concept coding and value coding (Saldaña, 2016), our chapter demonstrates how universities create complex discourses around mental health that, on one hand, normalize and destigmatize mental health, but on the other hand, prioritize student productivity as a primary impetus for mental health services while side-stepping institutional accountability for perpetuating ableist structures.

Literature Review: Coding Web 2.0 Resources in Health Rhetoric

We write alongside health rhetoric scholars who have already theorized methods of coding and understanding public-facing health resources. As J. Blake Scott and Lisa Melonçon (2017) have noted, because rhetoric of health and medicine scholarship tends to take on "complex, high-stakes phenomena," the use of mixed methodologies dominates much of the research in this field of inquiry (p. 4). Our project specifically takes up Judy Segal (2005)'s inquiry into "prior questions," or lines of inquiry that account for how providers, patients, and publics arrive at certain junctures; the prevailing assumptions, beliefs, and ideologies that regulate actions; and the operating practices that regulate interactions (p. 144). As Scott and Melonçon (2017) described it, research into prior questions of the rhetoric of health and medicine require researchers to "take a step back from the procedural questions typically posed by health and medicine experts to inquire about what makes certain meanings possible in the first place" (p. 5). To this end, this chapter utilizes textual analysis of various universities' public-facing counseling and mental health pages on their websites in order to interrogate how US institutions of higher education rhetorically construct mental health.

We consider these pages to be important research sites when trying to understand how universities construct mental health rhetorics and rich sites for furthering research in Health 2.0 because these sites have the potential to construct discourses of mental health that either support students in seeking help or reify stigmas and myths related to mental health. At the same time, these articulations of mental health express institutional responsibilities. Health 2.0 represents the many ways that individuals and communities are using networked sites and technologies for health-related purposes (Opel, 2017). Part of the development of Health 2.0 stems from the proliferation of texts related to mental health issues.

J. Fred Reynolds, David Mair, and Pamela Fischer (2013) noted that the "stigma-reducing 'treatable disorder' movement" has developed a snowball effect on textual production related to mental health issues throughout the past 20 years (p. 30). As conditions become seen as treatable, a flurry of textual production is set into motion: individuals seeking treatment for such conditions are seen in doctors' offices, instigating various texts, insurance companies development codes, explanation of benefits, and other documentation related to treatment, and the medical communities more broadly develop various texts in response to such conditions (Reynolds, Mair, & Fischer, 2013, pp. 30–31).

Universities participate in Health 2.0 by providing online spaces for students to locate mental health resources and, in so doing, frame the university's position on mental health. They often also offer clinical services for students. As M. Remi Yergeau and Bryce Heubner (2017) have argued, "how we filter information matters" (p. 279). Universities' online framings of mental health are cultivated through the twin processes of "filtering" the information they choose to represent on their websites and the information that is omitted (Yergeau & Heubner, 2017, p. 279). In the era of Web 2.0, when so many students seek answers and resources online, it is important to consider how universities participate in the creation and circulation of mental health information, a process which can rhetorically construct students' understanding of mental health and institutional responsibility in matters of mental health. We apply rhetorical scrutiny to these constructions in an effort to advocate for less ableist, more equitable institutional orientations toward mental health.

Methods: Coding Mental Health Rhetorics

Because we wanted to combine close, textual analysis of individual institutions' pages with an analysis of the various trends and patterns that appear among colleges and universities within the United States, we chose to build a corpus of university web pages that drew from various institution types. We specifically sought different types of institutions, such as two-year and four-year institutions, and public and private colleges and universities. We additionally wanted to pay attention to institutions with different student demographics, leading us to search for historically Black colleges and universities (HBCUs), Tribal colleges, Hispanic serving institutions (HSIs), and primarily white institutions (PWIs)[1] (see Table 11.1 below). We also consciously worked to gather institutions from various regions of the United States, with a total of 32 states represented in the corpus. Our goal in cataloging various institution types and states/regions prior to data analysis (beyond ensuring that we were including schools that served minoritized populations) was also to limit any unintentional bias or cherry-picking of institutions that might fit into the larger themes we saw emerging or excluding institutions that didn't meet our expectations.

TABLE 11.1 Classification of Universities for Website Corpus

HBCU 4-year public	HBCU 4-year private	HBCU 2-year public
HSI 4-year public	HSI 4-year private	HSI 2-year public
Tribal 4-year public	Tribal 2-year private	Tribal 2-year public

Our inclusion criteria were primarily based on demographic data. We used lists generated by the US Department of Education to locate his, HBCU, and Tribal universities and, from there, attempted to gather institutions from as many different states or regions as possible. Given that "PWI" is not an official designation used by the US Department of Education (Bourke, 2016), we created our lists of PWIs by attempting to determine which regions or states were not yet represented in our corpus, and then locating PWIs based on student demographic data provided on the institutions' websites. We excluded any institution for which we could not reasonably identify clear student demographic data or institutions that had no web pages related to mental health available to the public.

Based on these inclusion and exclusion criteria, we catalogued and coded four university websites for each institution type with two exceptions. First, we were only able to locate three private four-year Tribal colleges. Second, we were only able to catalog two two-year institutions in each institution type as outlined in Table 11.1 below, for a total of 39 university websites (fully itemized in Appendix A).

Because our primary interest was in how universities construct mental health, we applied concept coding and values coding to the data in our corpus. The first, concept coding, is used to determine how specific words and phrases contributed to a broader construction of a more abstract idea, such as mental health (Saldaña, 2016, pp. 119–120). With this round of coding, we were able to ask questions about how universities define mental health within their institutional spaces. We next coded the websites with value coding, which complements concept coding by analyzing what values, attitudes, and beliefs the universities embody within these textual sites (Saldaña, 2016, pp. 131–132). Together, concept and value coding helped us to understand how these mental health resource pages create and reify particular cultural assumptions and values about mental health.

Through these multilayered analyses, we found that universities create complex discourses around mental health that, on one hand, normalize and destigmatize mental health, but, on the other hand, prioritize student productivity as a primary impetus for mental health services. In so doing, our chapter illuminates not only "the values [universities] think about" but also "the values [universities] think *with*" (Segal, 2005, p. 119). More than simply understanding what universities say *about* mental health, our coding reveals how these institutions rhetorically construct mental health, how they frame their own institutional responsibility in mental health, and how these rhetorical constructions situate students.

The decision to sample four university websites, where possible, for each category was intended to aid us in achieving data saturation, which is generally defined as the point at which adding additional items for analysis (in this case, additional university websites to our corpus) no longer offers new information (Guest, Bunce, & Johnson, 2006). In the context of qualitative research involving coding, data saturation is achieved when no additional themes or coding emerge from the data set (Fusch & Ness, 2015). We found that no new coding themes were arising from the websites prior to coding the fourth website in each category (see Appendix B for the full list of codes), which led us to believe that data saturation had been achieved and that adding additional websites to our corpus and coding them would not lead us to any new codes or insights with regards to our research questions.

Findings and Analysis: Academic Success, Mental Health Pathologization, and Institutional Passivity

Through coding these institutional public-facing resources, we were able to conduct a textual analysis to better understand how this university sponsored rhetorical project functions on an institutional level. We used this textual analysis to understand the undercurrents of the rhetoric of mental health in this corpus of materials, much like Catherine Prendergast's (2001) textual analysis of the *DSM IV*, about which she argued that moving away from descriptivism functions to deny the rhetorical agencies of mad subjects (p. 54). We recognize that mental health services on campuses face a number of complicated challenges. Nevertheless, we echo Margaret Price's (2011) call that "It is crucial to understand psychiatric discourse *as* a rhetorical endeavor, not least because this discourse often claims to operate in ways that transcend rhetorical concerns such as context and audience" (p. 33). Our coding revealed a deep investment in academic success over well-being, an ableist pathologization of mental health, and a consistent use of passive language that functioned to distance institutions of postsecondary education from responsibility (especially highlighted in lukewarm statements about racial trauma). Below, we share these results and offer illustrative examples for each category of our findings.

Finding #1: University Mental Health Care for You(r) (Academic Success)

When we coded for the values universities communicate regarding providing mental health resources or the value of students seeking mental health resources, the most frequently communicated value was students' academic success. Of the 39 websites we coded, 18 of them, representing 46% of the corpus, emphasized that mental health resources could lead to increased academic success. Frequently, websites that reduced counseling to a means to academic success were framed in statements such as :"The Counseling Center helps students, undergraduate and graduate, achieve academic success" (University of Alabama, n.d.); counseling "Supports the institutional mission to graduate students" (Bowie State University, n.d.); counseling services are meant to address student concerns "that could impede their ability to achieve academically" (Lincoln University, n.d.); and that counseling centers are in place to assist students with personal issues that might "impact [your] college success" (Bishop State, n.d.).

The value of student successes emerges in each website in passages that directly address the mission of the counseling center and/or the part of the counseling websites in which the university communicates the purpose of the service. For example, Calumet College of Saint Joseph's Counseling Center states that "The SAP program is a free confidential counseling service provided to CCSJ students for personal and school concerns that may be interfering with academic performance and/or quality of life" (n.d.) Likewise, Arizona Western College includes the following language under the header that says "Services": "The office of Health and wellness exists to support students and their success. We are here to help students achieve their academic goals by encouraging a balance of health and well-being" (n.d.). We do not find it coincidental that universities signal student success in these places. The mission statement or explanations of the centers' roles are opportunities for universities to explain why particular services exist on campus. These statements provide a rationale for the existence of services. We find similarities in these mission statements or explanations of services as serving similar functions to the charter documents that have been so widely studied in technical communication (Dreher, 2017; Jones, 2018; McCarthy, 1991; McCarthy & Gerring, 1994). As explained by Lucille Parkinson McCarthy (1991) in her work on the *DSM-III*, and later in McCarthy & Gerring (1994), a charter document:

> establishes an organizing framework that specifies what is significant and draws people's attention to certain rules and *relationships* [emphasis added]. In other words, the charter defines as authoritative certain ways of seeing and deflects attention from other ways. It thus stabilizes a particular reality and sets the terms for future discussion.
>
> *(1991, p. 359)*

McCarthy's attention to how these documents establish and reify relationships among participants within a group helps us to understand what kinds of relationships universities are cultivating with students when they employ student success as the value of offering mental health resources. Within these framings, we see universities justifying the presence of mental health resources as tools that serve to fulfill universities' larger *a priori* goal of successfully graduating students.

The institutional values apparent in overpromotion of student success as the primary value for mental health resources are often coupled with passive statements about the difficulty of college. This trend is manifested in multiple codes from the corpus: seven websites (18%) conceptually constructed mental health concerns as arising because college is generally a time of stress and/or transformation. This concept code can be found in phrasing like "sometimes the demands of college life can seem stressful or overwhelming" (Alabama State, n.d.) or pointing to the "pressures that inevitably come with academic life" (Southwestern Christian College, n.d.). Sometimes, this passive language was also explicitly tied to student success, as in "difficult situations can get in the way of academic success" (St. Philip's College, n.d.).

In locating the impetus for mental health care in student's academic success, counseling centers reify a call to *normalcy*, ignoring how those same markers of academic success are ableist constructs (Dolmage, 2017; Price, 2011). This repeated framing of mental health issues as the obstacle to student success casts the university or college as a benevolent intercessor while refusing to address higher education's role in creating barriers for those who may be seeking mental health counseling, particularly neurodivergent or disabled individuals.

It's important to recognize that we do not necessarily believe that this attitude is shared by counselors and mental health experts working within any given university counseling center. Further research into mental health communication in higher education might consider who, for example, develops the materials on counseling pages and which governing bodies determine what content should be communicated. Nonetheless, our research has brought an important question to the surface: who is the intended audience of these statements? Or, in other words: for whom are these statements written and shared on counseling websites? We are concerned with how students understand their relationships with counseling centers and universities when the centers' goal is framed around academic success over or alongside their well-being.

While it may seem like emphasizing student success within university mental health resources is a natural consequence of the institutional hierarchy of university offices, we look to other counseling web pages from our corpus that deflect academic success as a value of mental health resources by invoking other values, such as improving students' quality of life, personal development, healing, and improving overall health. For example, University of California, Merced identifies the role of the counseling center as assisting student in achieving their own goals for themselves:

> Our goal is to help you identify YOUR goals. Then we work together to figure out what's been keeping you from achieving those goals and what

changes you can make in your life to be more successful in the future. We
encourage you to contact us with any concerns you may have.

(n.d., emphasis is original)

While the mission of this counseling center still invokes language around
"achievement," the emphasis on students' definition of what kind of development they want to pursue is a significant reframing. Similarly, University of
Houston, Clear Lake defines their goal around students' personal development:
"Counseling Services is committed to providing services in the best interest
of your emotional and mental health needs and continued personal growth"
(n.d.). As charter documents, these mission statements identify vastly different
sets of relationships between the counseling centers and students than universities that center academic success as the value of providing counseling services.
In mission statements/statements of services that focus on personal development, we see the centers promoting relationships with students that place students at the helm of their experiences at the counseling center. By encouraging
students to identify their own goals, counseling centers that privilege student
agency prioritize students' needs rather than the university's agenda for student
retention and success.

Finding #2: The Neuromyths Persist, or Pathologizing Mental Health

Through both our value and concept coding, a consistent pattern of the pathologizing of mental health emerged. By pathology, we mean the appeal to a
supposed "normative" mental state that certain people somehow transgress.
We see the pathologization of mental health emerge in the corpus of university
websites through several different concept codes. Ten web pages (representing
25% of the corpus), for example, placed an emphasis on mental health screenings and tests.

Moreover, in terms of concept coding, pathology frequently appeared in
treating mental health services as triage or emergency services; counseling centers become a place for when something *goes wrong*, for when mental health somehow diverges from the supposed normate (found in 24 websites, representing
61% of the corpus websites[2]). For example, Clemson University's web banner,
"do you feel ☹" pathologizes emotions of sadness by suggesting that students
should not, in fact, "feel ☹,"and that counseling might correct this[3] (n.d.).
These web documents consistently stressed the importance of "seeking help,"
a rhetorical framing that pathologizes those who seek counseling services by
constructing them as nonnormative, as "mentally unhealthy" (Dolmage, 2017,
p. 57). We echo Stella Akua Mensah and Stefanie Lyn Kaufman-Mthimkulu
(2020) here, who argued that "the notion of 'mental illness' was invented to
pathologize logical responses to the stress and trauma that are omnipresent in
a world brutalized by colonialism and capitalism" (n.d.). This pathologization

continues to adversely impact disabled people and, in particular, BIPOC disabled people. While we maintain that the idea of an ideal mental state is itself a neuromyth (Cedillo, 2018; Dolmage, 2014; Kafer, 2013; Moeller, 2014; Price, 2011; Yergeau, 2017), we note the persistence of this pathologized characterization in these institutional web pages.

Our concept coding revealed that, tethered to this rhetorical pathologizing of mental health for some (8 websites, representing 20% of the corpus) of these institutions, there was also an emphasis on "short-term" therapy.[4] Nineteen of the thirty-nine websites (48%) emphasized DIY approaches to mental health care for students, which included guides and readings on at-home mental health practices, links to external web resources, access to outsourced community-based or private mental health resources, and even social media platforms for peer support.

While counseling centers' resources are undoubtedly stretched thin, and while emergency mental health interventions are necessary, our concern is that this rhetorical framing of university mental health care as a short-term service may further stigmatize those who may require more sustained mental health care. Moreover, the move toward short-term counseling services appears to be connected to the larger project of neoliberalism on university campuses. As Bradley Lewis (2017) demonstrated, in the late 1980s there was a shift in how institutions of higher education dealt with mental health on their campuses. Prior to this time, universities tended to handle counseling and mental health resources by focusing on humanistic models that primarily addressed young adult development issues (p. 193). By the late 1980s, however, universities began adopting medical models of mental health, in which psychiatrists played larger roles, resulting today in more and more students "leav[ing] counseling centers with psychiatric disorders and medication as a key feature of their care" (Lewis, 2017, pp. 193–194). Coupled with the prevailing theme in these documents of "mental health for academic success," then, this pathologizing of mental health further obfuscates the ableism in postsecondary education: if you aren't attaining "academic success," the problem may be explained (blamed) on student mental health problems and *not* the ableism of postsecondary institutions, which creates barriers for those with mental health conditions. This rhetorical construction itself is an artificial barrier to addressing ableist structures that govern these institutions by framing the institution as a kindly intercessor in mental health concerns.

Finding #3: Mental Health from the "Outside" and Institutional Passivity

Another ten websites (25%) utilize language that identifies universities and colleges as passive forces within the context of students' mental health; they conceptually create mental health concerns as arising "outside" the institution in students' lives, as opposed to recognizing that universities often contribute to, inflame, or even create mental health concerns for students. In these examples, university websites recognize that "school concerns ... may be interfering with academic performance and/or quality of life" (Calumet College, n.d.) or suggest that "occasionally, students may encounter difficulties which challenge their coping skills and undermine their success in academic and personal endeavors" (College of Southern Idaho, n.d.). In one example, the site explains: "Difficult situations can get in the way of academic success" and then lists "anxiety, depression, loss of a relationship and other mental health-related issues" (St. Phillips, n.d.). In other words, students may experience mental health concerns, but these concerns apparently originate *off-campus*, not as a product of students' experiences at universities. These passive phrasings distance and insulate institutions from critique while obfuscating the barriers institutions create, placing the burden of "academic success" on the student seeking mental health counseling, and, importantly, ignoring how these same institutional structures may create or exacerbate mental health concerns and create barriers to academic success.

Moreover, the repeated rhetoric of the benevolent intercessor helping students achieve academic success ignores institutional culpability in exacerbating mental health concerns and the institutional barriers preventing academic success for those seeking mental health counseling to begin with. In short, these programs confuse university sanctioned markers of productivity (such as grades and attendance) not only as markers of mental health, but as *the goal* of mental health interventions.

This institutional passivity is echoed in responses to racism and racial violence: Since we were gathering our corpus as Black Lives Matter protests surged throughout the country following the tragic murders of George Floyd, Breonna Taylor, Ahmaud Abery, and others, our value and concept coding also turned toward an array of statements either expressing solidarity with students of color or expressing a commitment to addressing racial trauma. Seven of the websites we collected (18%) included statements affirming support for students of color and connecting racial violence to mental health. These statements themselves are important. Too often, racial trauma is not addressed, and those who claim to work on behalf of—and frequently speak for—marginalized people "will avoid the complexities of intersecting lives" (Brown, 2017, p. 1). Rhetorically, these statements from higher education counseling mimic the same patterns of institutions-as-benevolent framework we've described previously. In statements like "we recognize the detrimental impact that racism and any form of prejudice and discrimination have on mental health and well-being," (Northwestern, n.d.) and "CCS [Counseling and Consultation Service] acknowledges the impact on Ohio State students and recognizes that direct exposure to such violence can be traumatizing and result in emotional reactions," (The Ohio State, n.d.), we see similarities in passive phrasing.

These framings do not address how, for many students, these same academic institutions reinscribe racial traumas and are laden with racist policies. Furthermore, these statements on racial trauma ignore the relationship between racism, eugenics, and psychiatric study (Harbour et al., 2017; Tucker, 2005), just as disability studies too frequently ignores racial intersectionality (Annamma, Connor, & Ferri, 2013, p. 2013; Ben-Moshe & Magaña, 2014; Schalk, 2013). Our data analysis leads us to argue that rhetorical framings of racial trauma and mental health must undergo intersectional analysis while being critical of institutional culpability and simultaneously avoiding specifying action to address racism on their campuses—or even acknowledging the existence of racism on their campuses.

Conclusion: "How Do You Feel?" Reclaiming Institutional Responsibility for Equitable, Accessible Resources

Through concept and value coding, we did glimpse rhetorical constructions of mental health that were more inclusive and antiableist, and in working toward a conclusion, we look at how universities might reconstruct mental health more equitably. Building on the work that Barbara George and Rachel Blasiman (2021) do in their chapter in this volume, we extend concerns over whether or not college students know about and use the resources available to them to consider what messages students get about mental health in such resources. We have argued that university mental health must be more than institutional PR, and it must be pursued with equity, inclusion, and accessibility in mind, not merely retrofitted. To do this, we point to the rhetorical construction of mental health in the public-facing resources presented by Bowie State University, a public four-year HBCU. Their Counseling Center integrates access and contact with counseling services throughout students' degree programs, as part of a Four-Year-Experience Counseling Program. The Counseling Center's web page identifies their role first and foremost as supporting students "in their personal and psychosocial growth,"—a construction that moves away from a medical model of mental health, reminiscent of the preneoliberal constructions of counseling identified by Lewis (2017) (Bowie State University, n.d.). As presented in the material we collected, Bowie State's counseling program begins with a required Freshman Seminar course, taught by counselors. This course focuses, in part, on introducing students to the resources available on campus. Additionally, each year of a student's undergraduate program includes an interview with a counselor to identify and address "personal, social, career, and academic counseling" (Bowie State University, n.d.). The university derives the purpose of this program "from the belief that every student has basic and unique needs which must be fulfilled in order to function successfully in a learning environment" (Bowie State University, n.d.).

We see many opportunities emerging in Bowie State's representations of mental health more broadly, and the role of counseling and mental health services more specifically on their campus. The university's stated belief that students have basic needs related to mental health support runs contrary to the overwhelming trend of identifying counseling services and mental health resources as ad hoc crisis management. This move, in turn, rhetorically constructs mental health as the university's responsibility, rather than relying on the myth that disability more broadly (and mental health more specifically) is an individual's problem. Here we echo and amplify "Access is Love," a disability activist effort by Alice Wong, Mia Mingus, and Sandy Ho (2019)—three disabled Asian Americans who have insisted that "access should be a collective responsibility instead of a sole responsibility placed on a few individuals." In working to provide more thorough access, Bowie State's program (or at least how this program is described in their own public-facing resources—works to make mental health care a collective effort rather than a burden placed on the pathologized few who seek these services.

As rhetoricians interested in mental health rhetoric, we seek to intervene in the rhetorical project that frames the university as mental health champion while placing the onus of mental health care *on* its students, ignoring the institutional role sites of postsecondary education play in contributing to and exacerbating anxiety, depression, and other mental health concerns while minimizing a need for institutional change. As we work to better understand how these institutions rhetorically represent mental health in ways that frequently create barriers for disabled people, we also imagine how we may articulate mental health needs differently, radically refigured through a disability justice orientation, which—in the words of disability justice collective Sins Invalid (2019)—"names ableism as a constructed, violent ordering of bodily difference that our movement works to unmask and undo but it also recognizes that we currently exist in the world as it has been structured by ableism" (p. 65). We labor to hold institutions accountable for their ableist constructs and work toward the dream of a disability justice-oriented model of mental health: "as disabled people, we know that one of our biggest gifts is the Mad, sick, disabled, Deaf dreams we are always dreaming and have always been dreaming, way beyond what we are allowed to dream." (Piepzna-Samarasinha, 2020, p. 253).

While our analysis revealed problematic ideological and rhetorical framings, we find those framings that ran counter to neoliberal, pathologizing discourses to be more inclusive and just—like Bowie State's Freshman Seminar course mentioned above. Throughout our findings is a consistent thread: that university websites frame institutions of postsecondary education as benevolent institutions interceding in pathologized "crises" of mental health—all while distancing themselves from conversations about how these same institutions uphold systemic inequalities and policies harmful to student mental health. Rhetorically, these sites consistently read like public relations campaigns on behalf of their respective institutions. The rhetorical project represented in these documents, thus, reflects ableist understandings of mental health, which contribute to "the construction of a rigid, elitist, hierarchical and inhumane academic system" (Price, 2011, p. 8). Mental health resources are not exceptions to the pervasive ableism of higher education that function along with other interlocking systems of oppression to keep disabled people out—especially multiply marginalized disabled people. This chapter has attempted to use mental health rhetoric to intervene in these ableist constructions of mental health that sidestep institutional accountability.

APPENDIX A

List of Websites Analyzed

Hispanic-Serving Institutions (HSIs)

Public 4-Year Institutions

Kean University (New Jersey)
   Nyack College (New York)
   University of California, Merced (CA)
   University of Houston, Clear Lake (TX)

Private 4-Year Institutions

Calumet College of St. Joseph (IN)
   Carlos-Albizu University-Miami (FL)
   Heritage University (WA)
   University of the Southwest (NM)

Two-Year Public Institutions

Arizona Western College (AZ)
   Bakersfield College (CA)
   Morton College (IL)
   Norco College (CA)

Historically Black Colleges and Universities (HBCU)

Public 4-Year Institutions

Alabama State University (AL)
   Bowie State University (MD)
   Lincoln University (PA)
   Wilberforce University (OH)

Private 4-Year Institutions

Clinton College (SC)
   Edward Water College (FL)
   Howard University (DC)
   Southwestern Christian College (TX)

Two-Year Public Institutions

Bishop State Community College (AL)
   Coahoma Community College (MS)
   Southern University of Louisiana, Shreveport (LA)
   St. Philips College (TX)

Primarily White Institutions (PWI)

Four-Year Public Institutions

Clemson University (SC)
   Montana State University (MT)
   Ohio State University (OH)
   University of Alabama (AL)

Four-Year Private Institutions

Baylor University (TX)
   Georgetown (DC)
   Hamilton College (NY)
   Northwestern College (IL)

Two-Year Public Institutions

College of Southern Idaho (ID)
   Dyersburg State Community College (TN)
   Great Basin College (NV)

Tribal Institutions

Four-Year Public Institutions

Dine College (AZ)
   Haskell Indian Nations University (KS)
   Ilisagvik College (AK)
   Sinte Gleska University (SD)

Four-Year Private Institutions

College of Menominee Nation (WI)
   Turtle Mountain Community College (ND)
   United Tribes Technical College (ND)

Two-Year Public Institutions

Black Feet Community College (MT)
   Cankdeska Cikana Community College (ND)
   Fond Du Lac Tribal & Community College (MN)
   Keweenaw Bay Ojibwa Community College (MI)

APPENDIX B

Table of Value and Concept Codes with Corpus Frequencies Listed in Descending Order from Most Prevalent to Least Prevalent

Value Codes

The codes below represent what the websites depict as the value of providing mental health resources or students seeking mental health resources.

Code	Frequency	Percentage of Websites in Corpus (n = 39)
Students' academic success	18	46
Affordability (free, low-cost)	17	43
Personal development	14	35
Confidentiality, also HIPPA compliance	11	28
Inclusivity, multiculturalism, diversity	11	28
Students feeling supported	8	20
Students feeling safe	6	15
Healing	5	12
Mental health resources as part of the social justice mission of the university	5	12
Overall health	3	7
Quality of life	3	7
Economic achievement by staying in school	1	2
Citizen, global citizen	1	2

Concept Codes

The codes below represent how the universities framed the idea of mental health more broadly, rather than a specific resource, user, location, behavior, or technique.

Code	Frequency	Percentage of Websites in Corpus (n = 39)
Triage urgent crises (including suicide, after-hours resources)	24	61
DIY mental health resources (also "at home" resources, outsourced resources)	19	48
Peer support training/tools, group workshops	12	30
Sexual assault	11	28

(Continued)

Code	Frequency	Percentage of Websites in Corpus (n = 39)
Institution as passive force: mental health is something that exists "out there," rather than something universities create, inflame, or contribute to	10	25
Testing/Screening	9	23
Drug, Alcohol addictions/abuse	8	20
Normalized (mental health experiences are a normal part of peoples' lives)	8	20
Short-term mental health resources/ Intervention-oriented support	8	20
Racism, Racial Violence	7	18
College as stressful time/transformation	7	18
Developmental model of mental health (mental health issues are part of young adults' developmental processes)	6	15
Oriented around students' goals, student centered	6	15
Commonality: many students experience mental health	5	12
Wellness	5	12
Pathologization of mental health	2	5
Stigma, Mental health as stigmatized identity or experiences	2	5
Balance, well-balanced lives/behaviors	1	2
Seeking mental health help as a 'mature' response	1	2
Dignity	1	2

Notes

1 We are drawing upon M. Christopher Brown III and T. Elon Dancy II's (2010) definition of PWI's as institutions "in which Whites account for 50% or greater of the student enrollment" (p. 523). We located HBCU's through the US Department of Education's College Navigator website, and HSI's were located through the US Department of Education's Office of Postsecondary Education (OPE) fiscal year 2016 report of HSI's.

2 The triage concept code was the most prevalent code between the value and concept code.

3 We want to emphasize here that we are not opposed to students—or any individual, for that matter—seeking support from any mental health professional with or without diagnoses. Between the co-authors, we have multiple mental health diagnoses and respect each individual's ability to build a care plan that fits their needs. At the same time, however, we challenge what we see as a trend among university websites that pathologize and, in so doing, fix fluid embodied experiences in order to attempt to "correct" them.

4 We also find it significant to note that none of the websites specifically articulated commitments to long-term support. We recognize that this does not mean that universities do not have the resources or commitments to long-term infrastructures, but simply that universities do not actively construct their resources as such.

References

Annamma, Subini, Connor, David, & Ferri, Beth. (2013). Dis/ability critical race studies (DisCrit): Theorizing at the intersections of race and disability. *Race Ethnicity and Education, 16*(1), 1–31. https://doi.org/10.1080/13613324.2012.730511.

Ben-Moshe, Llat, & Magaña, Sandy. (2014). An introduction to race, gender, and disability: Intersectionality, disability studies, and families of color. *Women, Gender, and Families of Color, 2*(2), 105–114. doi:10.5406/womgenfamcol.2.2.0105.

Bourke, Brian. (2016). Meaning and implication of being labelled a primarily-white institution. *College and University, 91*(3), 12–21.

Bowie State University. (n.d.). *Counseling services.* Bowie State University. https://www.bowiestate.edu/campus-life/health-and-wellness/counseling-services/.

Brown, Lydia X. Z. (2017). Introduction: Notes from the field (not the ivory tower). In Lydia X. Z. Brown, E. Ashkenazy, and Morénike G. Onaiwu (Eds.), *All the weight of our dreams: On living racialized autism* (pp. 1–10). DragonBee Press.

Brown, M. Christopher, & Dancy, T. Elon. (2009). Predominantly white institutions. In Kofi Lomotey (Ed.), *Encyclopedia of African-American education* (pp. 523–526). https://www.doi.org/10.4135/9781412971966.n193.

Cedillo, Christina V. (2018). What does it mean to move? Race, disability, and critical embodiment pedagogy. *Composition Forum, 39.* https://compositionforum.com/issue/39/to-move.php.

Clemson University. (n.d.). *Counseling and psychological services.* Clemson University. https://www.clemson.edu/campus-life/student-health/caps/

Dolmage, T. Jay. (2014). *Disability rhetoric.* Syracuse University Press.

Dolmage, T. Jay. (2017). *Academic ableism: Disability and higher education.* University of Michigan Press.

Dreher, Kira. (2017). Insider audiences and plain-language revision: A city charter case study. *IEEE Transactions on Professional Communication, 60*(4), 430–447. doi:10.1109/TPC.2017.2759578.

Fusch, Patricia I., & Ness, Lawrence R. (2015). Are we there yet? Data saturation in qualitative research. *The Qualitative Report, 20*(9), 1408–1416. http://www.nova.edu/ssss/QR/QR20/9/fusch1.pdf.

George, Barbara, & Blasiman, Rachel. (2021). Online university mental health tools: Definitions and narratives as interventions. In Lisa Melonçon and Cathryn Molloy (Eds). *Strategic interventions in mental health rhetoric* (p. xx). Routledge.

Georgetown University. (n.d.). *Counseling and psychiatric services.* Retrieved from https://studenthealth.georgetown.edu/mental-health/.

Guest, Greg, Bunce, Arwen, & Johnson, Laura. (2006). How many interviews are enough? An experiment with data saturation and variability. *Field Methods, 18*(1), 59–82. https://doi.org/10.1177/1525822X05279903.

Harbour, Wendy S., Boone, Rosalie, Bourne Heath, Elaine, & Ledbetter, Sislena G. (2017). "Overcoming" in disability studies and African-American culture: Implications for higher education. In Stephanie L. Kerschbaum, Laura T. Eisenman,

& James M. Jones (Eds.), *Negotiating disability: Disclosure and higher education* (pp. 149–170). University of Michigan Press.

Jones, Natasha N. (2018). Human centered syllabus design: Positioning our students as expert end-users. *Computers and Composition, 49,* 25–35. doi:10.1016/j.compcom.2018.05.002.

Kafer, Alison. (2013). *Feminist, queer, crip.* Indiana University Press.

Lewis, Bradley. (2017). Postmodern madness on campus: Narrating and navigating mental difference and disability. In Stephanie L. Kerschbaum, Laura T. Eisenman, & James M. Jones (Eds.), *Negotiating disability: Disclosure and higher education* (pp. 191–209). University of Michigan Press.

McCarthy, Lucille Parkinson. (1991). A psychiatrist using DSM-III: The influence of a charter document in psychiatry. In Charles Bazerman and James Paradis (Eds.), *Textual dynamics of the profession: Historical and contemporary studies of writing in professional communities* (pp. 358–378). University of Wisconsin Press.

McCarthy, Lucille Parkinson, & Gerring, Joan Page. (1994). Revising psychiatry's charter document: DSM-IV. *Written Communication, 11*(2), 147–192. doi:10.1177/07 41088394011002001.

Mensah, Stella, & Kaufman-Mthimkhulu, Stefanie L. (2020, July 22). *Abolition must include psychiatry.* Disability Visibility Project. https://disabilityvisibilityproject.com/2020/07/22/abolition-must-include-psychiatry/.

Moeller, Marie. (2014). Pushing boundaries of normalcy: Employing critical disability studies in analyzing medical advocacy websites. *Communication Design Quarterly, 2*(4), 52–80. https://doi.org/10.1145/2721874.2721877.

Northwestern. (n.d.) *Coping with recent events: CAPS statement against racism and police brutality.* Northwestern Counseling and Psychological Services. https://www.northwestern.edu/counseling/outreach-education/coping-with-recent-events/index.html.

Opel, Dawn. (2017). Ethical research in "Health 2.0": Considerations for scholars of medical rhetoric. In. J. Blake Scott & Lisa Melonçon (Eds.) *Methodologies for the rhetoric of health and medicine* (pp. 176–194). Routledge.

Piepzna-Samarasinha, Leah L. (2020). Still dreaming wild disability justice dreams at the end of the world. In Alice Wong (Ed.), *Disability visibility: First-person stories for the twenty-first century* (pp. 250–261). Vintage Books.

Prendergast, Catherine. (2001). On the rhetoric of mental disability. In James C. Wilson & Cynthia Lewiecki-Wilson (Eds.), *Embodied rhetoric: Disability in language and culture* (pp. 45–60). Southern Illinois University Press.

Price, Margaret. (2011). *Mad at school: Rhetorics of mental disability and academic life.* University of Michigan Press.

Reynolds, J. Fred, Mair, David C., & Fischer, Pamela C. (2013). *Writing and reading mental health records: Issues and analysis in professional writing and scientific rhetoric.* Routledge. doi:10.4324/9780203811221.

Saldaña, Johnny. (2016). *The coding manual for qualitative researchers* (3rd ed.). SAGE.

Schalk, Sami. (2013). Coming to claim crip: Disidentification with/in disability studies. *Disability Studies Quarterly, 33*(2). http://dx.doi.org/10.18061/dsq.v33i2.3705.

Scott, J. Blake, & Melonçon, Lisa. (2017) *Methodologies for the rhetoric of health and medicine.* Routledge.

Segal, Judy. (2005). *Health and the rhetoric of medicine.* Southern Illinois University Press.

Sins Invalid. (2019). *Skin, tooth, and bone: The basis of our movement is our people* (2nd ed.). Sins Invalid.

St. Philip's College. (n.d.). *Counseling services.* St. Philip's College. https://www.alamo. edu/spc/experience-spc/current-students/safe-space/counseling-services/.

Tucker, William H. (2005). The racist past of the American psychology establishment. *The Journal of Blacks in Higher Education, 48,* 108–112. doi:10.2307/25073255.

University of Chicago. (n.d.). *Student health and counseling services.* University of Chicago. https://wellness.uchicago.edu/mental-health/.

Yergeau, M. Remi. (2017). *Authoring autism: On rhetoric and neurological queerness.* Duke University Press.

Yergeau, M. Remi, & Huebner, Bryce. (2017). Minding theory of mind. *Journal of Social Philosophy, 48*(3), 273–296. doi:10.1111/josp.12191

Wong, Alice, Mingus, Mia, & Ho, Sandy. (2019, Feb. 1). Access is Love [blog post]. Disability Visibility Project. https://disabilityvisibilityproject.com/2019/02/01/ access-is-love/.

12

ONLINE UNIVERSITY MENTAL HEALTH TOOLS

Definitions and Narratives as Interventions

Barbara George and Rachael Blasiman

Introduction

In their chapter, "Manifesting Methodologies for the Rhetoric of Health and Medicine," Blake Scott and Lisa Melonçon (2018) pointed to Ellen Barton's notion of "disciplined interdisciplinarity" as a suggestion for "...producing knowledge recognizable and valued by different scholarly areas (p. 314)" (p. 11). As the editors of this collection note, mental health concerns are complex in nature. We acknowledge this complexity in this chapter by working across disciplines, combining rhetorical and psychological research to explore the emerging practice of universities offering online mental health tools to students as interventions. In our chapter, we address two issues in mental health access. One concern is the low rate of mental health help-seeking among college students, while the other is the lack of research about how students actually make use of tools such as online resources. Since many universities are curating and creating resources for web-based or online mental health supports, we looked specifically at access to and persuasive messaging in online interventions. In our analysis, we paid particular attention to narratives and definitions found within online messaging as these might or might not lead students to find mental health resources online, or, through the online services, connect to in-person supports.

Specifically, our study examines ways that students engage with online mental health support tools offered at a small midwestern regional university. By investigating how students access and interact with these tools, our empirical research study considers how definitions of mental health and contextualizing narratives, whether in the tools themselves or offered as introductions to the tools, can serve as interventions. After analyzing our data, we ultimately argue

DOI: 10.4324/9781003144854-16

that universities' online mental health tools should be shared with students in more intentional ways—beyond providing a link to services that students are expected to navigate themselves.

Literature Review

This study enters into discussions of mental health rhetoric research (Reynolds, 2018) and connects to health scholarship that considers relationship between rhetoric and technical communication (Holladay, 2017; Melonçon & Frost, 2015). This research also intersects with health communication scholarship that highlights the importance of narrative in framing and communicating clinical health concerns (Charon, 2001).

University interventions are often the first mental health supports many students encounter as young adults. Moreover, while psychology scholarship acknowledges that university students experience high rates of mental health distress, it is recognized that university students often do not seek mental health support (Hartrey, Denieffe, & Wells, 2017). Students' perceptions of mental health supports are heavily influenced by how they are introduced to such supports, and when such introductions aren't handled carefully, barriers to mental health help-seeking behaviors can emerge. These barriers can include: students having no knowledge of services and/or how to access them; students avoiding support due to stigma; and students' inability to identify a personal need for mental health support. Such barriers can be compounded by time constraints and institutional constraints (for example, student time constraints and institutional constraints like limited counseling resources). In response, there has been a push for alternative platforms to offer flexible support, such as virtual or online services (Farrer et al., 2015, pp. 1–2). Naturally, the push for more virtual and online services also increased rapidly due to the COVID-19 pandemic.

Other research on the topic of mental health resources for college students explores how universities have developed or invested in online mental health supports for students as interventions in an effort to end the stigma surrounding mental health and to encourage mental health help-seeking (Harrer at al., 2018). These supports, such as online screening tools and websites highlighting mental health issues and resources, have shown some promise in encouraging mental health help-seeking behaviors. For example, Mathias Harrer and colleagues' (2018) meta-analysis of 48 psychological studies of the effects that internet interventions have on university students' mental health found "small effects on depression, anxiety, and stress symptoms, as well as moderate-sized effects on eating disorder symptoms and students' social and academic functioning" (p. 14). Similarly, a recent study that consisted of small student focus groups found that virtual mental health clinics were viewed "favorably" by students—particularly those who might have avoided other types of intervention, such as face-to-face counseling, due to stigma (Farrer et al., 2015). Similarly, Megan Ryan, Ian Shochet, and Helen Stallman's 2010 study found that online access to mental health services can improve mental health help-seeking in terms of drastically higher numbers of students accessing supports: "Rates of access for student counselling services reported previously have been as low as 5% ... whereas this study found that almost 50% of students would use an online program..." (p. 81).

Despite these encouraging results, there are questions about how students access, perceive, and use online supports, resulting in calls for more research to further evaluate online mental health support tools offered by universities, particularly in terms of entry points into the use of the supports (Lattie, Lipson, & Eisenberg, 2019). Researchers have suggested that there are rhetorical choices that universities can adopt to make supports more accessible to students (Scholten & Granic, 2019). We argue that narrative framing and specific definitions of mental health are crucial parts of access and design within university communications about mental health. Understanding narrative framing, or the way mental health and mental health help-seeking are presented to or contextualized for students, is important in terms of how "stories" about mental health help-seeking are told, either by an instructor or counselor introducing the tools in real time, or on the site itself. Similarly, definitions of mental health that normalize mental health help-seeking might allow students to more easily choose a mental health intervention. Mindful approaches to both narrative framing and to crafting definitions of mental health, we argue, can lead to more effective interventions.

Description of Study

While university online tools are designed to intervene in cases of mental health distress, we believe that it is important to study how they do so rhetorically to understand the relationship between the intended message and the ways the audience perceives the message. We do so by first analyzing the online mental health tools themselves. Here, we explore patterns of persuasion, looking at the ways definitions and narratives on such sites "frame" mental health concepts.

Likewise, we examine students' interactions with online mental health interventions via focus groups. Focus group data illuminate audiences' perceptions of tool use, including whether different types of contextualizing narratives paired with online mental health tools impact students' emerging understanding of mental health definitions. Our findings suggest that students respond favorably to university tools introduced by instructors or counselors in a class setting—particularly when such persons can contextualize the tools; that resources should be repeatedly advertised in many contexts throughout the semester; that narratives about mental health can be helpful if they are relatable to students; and that links to human-centered supports (whether face-to-face or digital) should be clear and should emphasize confidentiality.

Rhetorical Analysis of Online Tools

In an effort to understand the means of persuasion in our university's online mental health tools, we describe rhetorical patterns found in the selected online tools our focus group students had access to. Because meta-analysis of digital mental health tools revealed that more work must be done to understand how student efficacy in mental health help-seeking behavior is linked to the design of the tools themselves (Scholten & Granic, 2019), we first analyzed the online tools offered to students to understand how definitions of mental health are constructed, and how narratives are used to encourage mental health help-seeking behavior. Since the university has dedicated considerable resources to these online supports, we began to consider several initial questions about if and how these online support services "worked" for our students. This initial analysis of the tools themselves later shaped our focus group research questions, which included:

- Do these tools refer to human-related services (such as speaking to a counselor), or are they designed to offer digital mental health supports as contained within the site itself?
- Are these sites introduced by an instructor in an introductory course (and, if so, did instructors play a role in students' understanding of these sites?))
- Do students navigate these sites on their own, or are they guided through sites?
- How do students react to the attempts at destigmatizing mental health help-seeking behaviors on these sites?
- Are there ways mental health definitions and narratives might be communicated to help students to recognize when seeking help might be appropriate?

Upon further review of the ways these sites could be "used," we were also aware that additional considerations, such as design, usability (how information is accessed), and how users navigate through information, create narratives, and inform definitions that might impact how students use these sites for mental health help-seeking. As we shared counseling pages with our students, more questions emerged. First, we wondered whether students were finding these online pages. Next, we wondered: when and if they did so, were they compelled to navigate through the site? Did they prefer to navigate through the site on their own, or with an instructor or advisor, and did guidance allow for a deeper understanding of mental health supports?

Before going further into our focus groups and findings, we want to discuss the specific mental health tools our study includes and to share how our questions for the focus groups deepened as we examined them. These tools can vary among institutions. We, thus, feel that a rich description of the tools used in our study is important for the understanding of our research design and focus group questions. Of particular importance to our study design was a desire to know how the students interpreted the messages of the tools, particularly in terms of possible shifts in the definition of mental health as well as in dispositions toward mental health stigma.

Description of Tools

On the university landing page offering counseling support to students, there are three columns. 24/7 emergency information is placed prominently on both the left and the right columns. These include, among other emergency supports, a nurse's hotline, a crisis text line, and the National Suicide Prevention Hotline. This repeated information is easy to find, though there is generally no context or descriptions beyond the contact numbers offered. We, thus, wondered: Would students understand when and how to use these resources? Less obvious is an online link to "Request Counseling Services" and information for "Counselor Contacts and Office Locations" through which students can arrange to meet with a local counselor. Thus, on the initial landing page, echoing findings in Leslie Anglesey and Adam Hubrig's study in this volume, much of the information frames mental health help-seeking in terms of responses to emergencies—an understandable feature as students may access the page when they are already in distress. This may, however, inadvertently send the message that counseling services are to be accessed in dire emergencies, muddying definitions of mental health and contributing to mental health stigma.

However, in the center column, but less prominently displayed, there is a shift to richer definitions of mental health concerns. A more contextualized paragraph, titled "COUNSELING HELPS" describes, using the first person, how counseling might be beneficial to students (see Figure 12.1).

In Figure 12.1, the unnamed speaker makes a connection with the audience in two ways. First, by stating "All of us can relate to those statements" in reference to counseling, the writer attempts to "normalize" counseling through the inclusive "us." Next, the writer points to interventions students may have already tried (speaking to friends or family), before suggesting another option—campus counseling, revealing the purpose of the message. After examining this tool, we wondered: Did attempts to normalize mental health through communicative moves impact how students might consider engaging in mental health supports beyond emergencies? This analysis led to specific questions in our focus group design.

Definition within Tools

As researchers, we also attended to concerns of "de-stigmatizing" mental health by exploring "definitions" to clarify how students' definitions of mental

COUNSELING HELPS

All of us can relate to those statements. Many times being able to talk it out can help. Many times we can talk it out with friends and family. And other times counseling is a useful and effective option. If your academic plan for success is out of balance due to any reason, consider counseling services. The services are free, safe, private and confidential. Our focus is your success at Kent State University and beyond. We promote prevention, education and personal empowerment through our educational and counseling services.

FIGURE 12.1 Counseling helps.

health might shift while engaging with online mental health tools. As our results show, working with the students interacting with tools during the focus groups helped us to understand how students' shifting definitions about mental health can coincide with their emerging sense of agency about mental health. Specifically, as students in our focus groups chose to identify and engage with, or reject, mental health concepts as presented in online tools, they clarified personal definitions of mental health.

Moreover, in designing our focus groups, we became aware of a pattern wherein tools are clearly designed to address low levels of mental health help-seeking behaviors by university students. For example, below the COUNSELING HELPS statement noted in Figure 12.1, there is a link titled "Services for Students" that, when selected, offers more specific reasons for counseling through a "Some Reasons for Counseling" section with which students might identify (see Figure 12.2). Here, specific feelings and scenarios (definitions) are described to more clearly link to "reasons for counseling" (actions), which can be accessed through counselor contact information on the previous page.

In Figure 12.2, several mental health issues are presented as reasons for counseling, such as "Feeling Overwhelmed, Stressed Out." As we analyzed these definitions listed on counseling sites, we wondered whether students might identify with these more specific reasons to attend counseling that they had

SOME REASONS FOR COUNSELING:

- Feeling Overwhelmed, Stressed Out
- Balancing School, Work and Family/Parenting
- Worry, Fear, Anxiousness, Shy
- Sadness, Moodiness, Irritable
- Anger, Conflict
- Difficulty Dealing with Grief or Any type of Loss
- Relationship, Parenting, Family and/or Work Issues
- Procrastination, Perfectionism
- Test Anxiety
- Self-Injury, Suicidal Thoughts
- Poor Time Management and/or Organization Skills
- Build Communication Skill, Self-Esteem, Confidence
- Addictions (gambling, spending, gaming, etc.)
- Alcohol or Drug Concerns (misuse, abuse)
- Bullying
- Sexual Identity
- Concerns about Life after Graduation

FIGURE 12.2 Some reasons for counseling.

not previously considered, potentially reaching out to counseling services—a consideration we added to our focus group questions.

There are tools that frame interventions in more clinical ways on the site. Below the "services" link, for instance, is a "Free Anonymous Mental Health Screening" tool (see Figure 12.3), Notably, this tool uses the term "mental health" for the first time on the site. The description of the link does not make clear who exactly the speaker is, or who or what method facilitates the "screening," but does offer discretion through the repeated term "anonymous."

The descriptor in Figure 12.3 employs clinical terms, which did not appear on the site before, such as "screening," "bi-polar disorder," and "PTSD." Unlike the list provided in Figure 12.2, where students could self-identify with a list to define mental health concerns, the screening tool is situated as an authority with "results" that link to campus counseling supports. The student becomes the recipient of a mental health definition as a result of a screening program in this scenario, which the student may or may not accept. A specific action, campus counseling, is suggested after viewing results. Since this is a more clinical approach to mental health help-seeking than the more colloquial definitions in Figure 12.2, we wanted to know the following through our focus

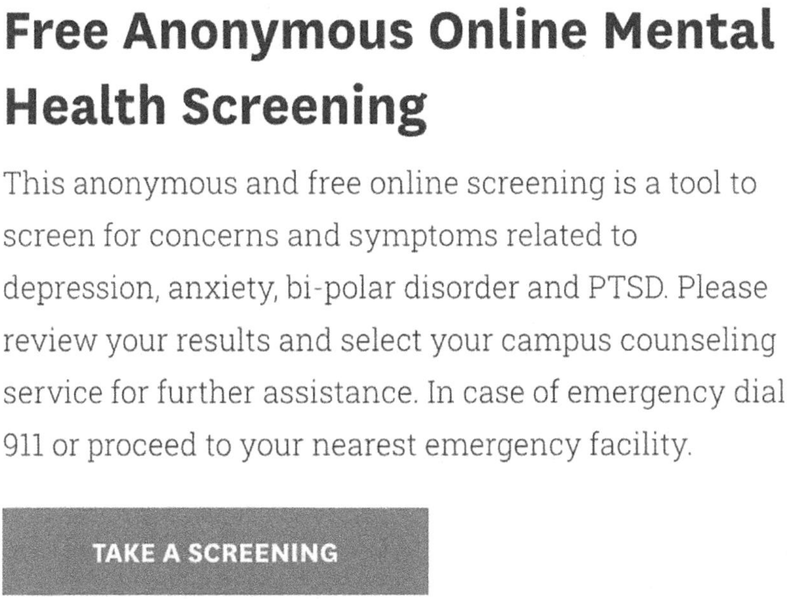

Free Anonymous Online Mental Health Screening

This anonymous and free online screening is a tool to screen for concerns and symptoms related to depression, anxiety, bi-polar disorder and PTSD. Please review your results and select your campus counseling service for further assistance. In case of emergency dial 911 or proceed to your nearest emergency facility.

TAKE A SCREENING

FIGURE 12.3 Free anonymous online mental health screening.

groups: Did this kind of framing, which appeared to be more clinical, impact students as they considered mental health supports? Or did the clinical framing of mental health inhibit mental health help-seeking?

Narratives within Tools

To extend the notion of shifting definitions of mental health that might normalize mental health help-seeking, we also explored the rhetorical considerations of storytelling or narratives and their capacity to build ethos with an audience. Rita Charon's (2001) discussions of narrative medicine in medical practice considered how narratives can improve discourse about public health. Renuka Uthappa (2017) explored the intersections of narrative, disability disclosure, and stigma, focusing on the benefits of mental disability disclosure despite its capacity to render the speaker vulnerable; storytelling can effectively challenge mental health stigma through the ethos of the speaker (pp. 173–174).

We were curious about the narratives embedded in the tools on our site and how students might or might not relate to them. One example of the textual and video narratives in the online university tools is found near the bottom of the site through a button that leads to a program called "Half of Us." The name itself, of course, could be read as a rhetorical choice intended to normalize mental health help-seeking behavior; as the page continues, "half of college students reporting that they have been stressed to a point where they couldn't function during the past year." After selecting this button, a user is taken to a page with a young, white, college-aged woman. Below her are the lines "Kortni Shares Her Story" followed by a narrative discussion of a television episode related to Kortni. Here, the mental health concerns and interventions are couched in a narrative. In the episode summary, Kortni's narrative establishes a concern— excessive drinking: "Kortni struggles with pain and anxiety connected to trauma in her past after a night of drinking." The drinking is a result of specific mental health precursors: trauma and anxiety. Kortni reaches out for support by "speaking to Dr. Drew" about the intertwined issues of trauma, anxiety, and drinking, eventually resulting in a "powerful impact [of] help-seeking." After her narrative, the paragraph shifts to addressing the audience directly to expand definitions of mental health concerns. Kortni's narrative attempts to offer a destigmatizing approach to trauma, anxiety, and alcohol use in an attempt to build ethos with a college-aged audience to encourage interventions. Our analysis of these narratives of college-aged individuals sharing their experience led us to ask, in our focus groups: Are these destigmatizing narratives with celebrities or on shows effective at encouraging mental health help-seeking behaviors among students?

The narratives on the site also act as a bridge to link to other tools on the site that offer even more links between definitions and interventions. For instance, a 24/7 number students can text and/or call offers immediate assistance immediately below the narrative. Other links appear as intertextual options on the landing page and other pages, solidifying the connection between defining a mental health issue and providing resources for concerns. For example, there are several ways to click to general definitions, such as a "Dealing With" button that leads to "I'm feeling" with options, and "I'm experiencing," which allows students to choose more options. The options are not clinical in nature, perhaps in an attempt to appeal to audiences for whom clinical descriptions would lead to increased stigma or at least to activation of existing stigmatized views. Students can self-identify through the "I'm" statements by clicking on an emotion, experience, or fact, which defines the concern in a general manner, then offers a "Feel Better option," which lists bulleted points for dealing with the emotion or situation, or a "Find Help Now" button, which links to general emergency supports (phone and text numbers for national hotlines). There are more "stories" linked throughout, usually video clips of celebrities sharing how they worked through a difficult personal event linked to emotions, experiences, or facts specific to what students may have self-selected. Throughout the site, there are many visuals of college-aged students discussing mental health or active in mental health campaigns and supports, again, an attempt to "normalize" mental health help-seeking. As we analyzed this approach to mental health interventions, we wanted to address the following questions in our focus group: Were students identifying with or rejecting these narrative and definitional online tools, or were descriptions of mental health supports given by instructors or mental health professionals more compelling for students?

While we described the design of many of the tools through our own analysis of them and used rhetorical analysis to guess at purpose and aim, we felt that it was vital to understand how students used and viewed the tools themselves. We, thus, used our analyses of the tools to generate a full list of question to consider in focus groups, and they are highlighted in the bulleted list below. We were particularly interested in learning more fully whether students' definitions might shift through tools, particularly through narratives. These, finally, are our focus group questions:

- Were students finding online mental health supports on their own?
- If they found the sites, were they compelled to navigate through the sites?
- Did they prefer to navigate the sites on their own, or with an instructor, counselor, or advisor?

  - Did human guidance through online features allow for a deeper understanding of mental health supports?

- How did design impact the way students "read" the sites?
- Did attempts to normalize mental health help-seeking through communicative moves (for example, by providing definitions or narratives) impact how students might consider engaging in mental health supports beyond emergencies?
- Did students identify with more specific reasons to attend counseling when they were provided with definitions and/or narratives that they had not previously considered—potentially leading to students being more willing to reach out to counseling services?
- Did clinical framings encourage or inhibit students as they considered mental health help-seeking?
- Are destigmatizing narratives with celebrities or with reality television personalities effective at encouraging mental health help-seeking behaviors?

  - Were students identifying with or rejecting these narratives?
  - Were descriptions of mental health supports given by instructors or university mental health professionals more compelling for students than these celebrity narratives?
  - Was a mixture of both celebrity and instructor/university mental health professionals effective?

Student Focus Groups

After approval from our university's Institutional Review Board,[1] we recruited students from our classes for our focus group study. Students were assured that participation was entirely voluntary, that there would be no penalty for choosing not to participate, and that their responses would be deidentified before analysis. We recruited students from two undergraduate classes during the spring 2020 semester and three more undergraduate classes in the fall 2020 semester. All five classes were roughly the same size (about 14 students), taught synchronously, and made up of students who were primarily in their first year of college. During the spring 2020 semester, seven students participated in the focus group sessions and 32 students participated in the fall 2020 semester focus groups.

Preintervention Resource Knowledge

All five classes were given the same baseline questions during the focus groups, before any campus resources were presented. These preintervention questions are listed in Table 12.1. We chose these questions to (a) better understand students' current level of resource knowledge and (b) assess their a priori perceptions of mental health stigma. Students could choose to answer these questions during the focus group or post them to a discussion board.

TABLE 12.1 Questions Used in Focus Groups

Questions asked before presentation

If a fellow student told you they needed to see a counselor, what would you tell them, or what supports would you direct them to?

Why do you think people who need mental health counseling resist getting help?

What are some of the things you hear people say about getting help for mental health concerns?

Questions asked after presentation

Were you aware that these resources existed before you were presented with them today? If so, who told you about them or how did you find about them?

What is the best/most helpful aspect of these resources to help you to understand mental health? What could improve the website for accessing support?

What could make resources better overall so that mental health supports can be more clear?

Do you think these tools could change the way some people who resists getting mental health support? Why or why not?

After viewing these resources, has your definition of mental health changed? If so, how?

Questions only for Narrative Group

How did reading/hearing stories of people dealing with mental health, whether in the online resources itself or in the introduction to the resources, impact your understanding to mental health?

Were there examples where reading/hearing stories of people dealing with health concerns did not align with your understanding of mental health?

How important do you think stories within the tools themselves are in helping students to understand mental health supports?

How important do you think stories provided before accessing tools are in helping students understand mental health supports?

I think people who need help are afraid of the backlash they will receive if they ask for help or recognize they are unhealthy in some way. I think a lot of people also get stuck in denial thinking they have it under control or that they are not sick.

I think people who need mental health counseling resist getting help because they are scared to admit that they need help or that people will make fun of them for going to counseling.

I believe people that need mental health counseling often times resist getting help because they do not want to accept the fact that they need help and also don't want the other people around them in their life to look at them any differently or treat them any differently because of it.

I feel like people resist getting help because they do not want to think that something is wrong with them, and they feel like they will be able to get better on their own. I also feel like they do not want their friends and family to look at them differently because they are seeking out help.

I think that people do not want to be seen as weak or damaged, so they 'tough it out' and do not get the help that they need.

FIGURE 12.4 Sample coding.

After all responses were submitted, we coded line-by-line for frequently occurring words and phrases, using grounded theory (Charmaz, 2006). These words and phrases were then tabulated and used to assess emerging themes. For example, in response to the question, "Why do you think people who need mental health counseling resist getting help," we found linguistic patterns that revealed how students understood stigma and mental health definitions, as is shown in the selection of responses in Figure 12.4.

Overall, our preintervention question responses revealed that students knew that mental health resources, which they identified as people or professionals they trusted, should be available to the public, but students did not know how to access university resources. In many cases, students did not know these university resources existed. In the spring 2020 semester, for example, we collected responses from seven students. Students were asked what they would do if they or someone close to them needed mental health support. One student responded, "...I would tell them to just talk to someone in their family." Another commented, "I would tell them to find a trusted adult to talk to." Two additional students agreed that they would "tell them to talk to someone in their family." Interestingly, both campus counselors were present in this online session while students responded to this question, but not one student said they would tell someone to go see a mental health counselor.

In the fall 2020 semester, we collected responses from 32 students on this same question. Unexpectedly, responses were quite different from the spring semester. The most common response (13 students) said they would see a counselor or therapist. In addition, 12 students said they would go online to find mental health resources, either "Googling symptoms" or searching for a local therapist. The third most common response, though, was more in line with the spring semester; students said they would go to their parents (eight students) or speak to some other trusted adult (four students). Eight students suggested they would talk to a friend. One student thought they would see their primary care doctor, one student said they would check with their health insurance provider, and one student said they had no idea where to turn if they needed mental health support. In a follow-up question, students were asked how they would advise a friend who came to them with mental health concerns. Students overwhelmingly replied that they would tell their friend to see a counselor (19 students) or speak to a parent/trusted adult (13 students).

We make two interesting observations about student responses to this preintervention question. First, in addition to differences in the number of students who volunteered to share their responses, there is a marked difference between spring 2020 and fall 2020 in actual student responses to our questions. In the spring, students did not even consider seeing a counselor for a mental health concern, but seeing a counselor was the number one response in the fall semester. One possible explanation for this difference is an increase in national messaging about mental health during the COVID-19 pandemic and a greater awareness of mental health issues related to quarantine, such as depression and anxiety.

A second interesting observation is the difference between what students would do themselves and what advice they would give to a friend. Their own actions seemed more varied and included more internet searching, but they would clearly tell a friend to see a counselor or speak to a trusted adult. However, and most importantly in terms of our study, they did not indicate the use of university tools in any scenario.

Preintervention Perceptions of Mental Health Stigma

In addition to knowledge of mental health resources, we also asked students for their perceptions of mental health issues. These responses highlighted ways students perpetuated or thwarted mental health help-seeking stigma. We asked students in the focus groups what they would tell a friend who was experiencing mental health issues. Nine students would tell a friend that they support them, nine students would tell a friend they are "there for them" or would "help in any way they could," and two students said they would simply "listen" to support their friend. Six students mentioned they would reassure a friend that "it's okay" and "not judge that they are going to a counselor" to seek help. Two students said they wouldn't know what to say.

We also asked our students for their opinions about why people resist getting therapy for mental health concerns. Students responded that people are ashamed or embarrassed (12 responses), scared/afraid (8 responses), or think "they can get through it on their own" (10 responses). They also think people feel judged (5 responses), are seen as weak (6 responses), or will be treated differently (3 responses). Several students suggested that some people are in denial about their problems (7 responses), don't realize they need help (3 responses), or don't know where to get help (2 responses). One student noted that, "some [people] don't know how dangerous it is to try to deal with things on their own." When asked what things they hear other people say about getting counseling, some students saw this as a "normal thing" while others said it "wasn't something people talked about." One student felt they had been forced into counseling in the past due to family concerns and resented their lack of agency in that decision. This student felt that all counseling should be a choice and that each person reacts to personal situations differently. These attitudes about mental health help-seeking, particularly in the context of designing tools that are responsive to perceived sigma and choice, are important in light of persuasive messaging that universities might consider.

Our Intervention

We designed two interventions to compare their efficacy at changing student knowledge about campus resources and improving knowledge of mental illness. The first, the Counselor Intervention, was a counselor-led session in which the campus counselor presented mental health resources. The second, the Narrative Intervention, was an instructor-led session in which the campus mental health website was presented, and students viewed several narrative videos provided as resources on the page. The instructor showed the students where the narratives were, but asked students to navigate the narrative sections themselves. Three classes (one in spring and two in fall) received the Counselor intervention and two classes (one in spring and one in fall) received the Narrative intervention.

We chose these two interventions for several reasons. First, both interventions are simple to implement. They both require little course preparation beyond reviewing the campus resources ahead of time or submitting a request to the campus counselor. Second, each of these interventions would be easy to replicate at other universities; nearly every university has a mental health presence online, and most have access to campus counselors. Third, we were curious if one intervention would be more effective than another—particularly considering how students might respond to the human-guided Counselor intervention versus the self-guided Narrative intervention. Comparing these two interventions directly would allow us to make this judgment.

After the intervention, all students in the focus groups were asked an additional series of questions (see Table 12.1) about their experience and potential use of these resources in the future. In addition, the Narrative group was asked supplementary questions about the stories they viewed (see Table 12.1 above).

Postintervention Responses: Counselor Group

For the spring 2020 Counselor group session, two campus counselors joined the online synchronous class and shared the campus mental health website, a presentation filled with local resources, and an online workbook specifically made for students experiencing anxiety and/or depression during the spring 2020 quarantine. This class was just beginning a unit on mental health, and the first lecture addressed issues of stigma, lifetime prevalence rates for mental illness, and clinical definitions of mental health. Students in the focus group were able to interact with both counselors throughout the session.

After the counselors concluded their presentation to the students, the instructor asked students to complete the postintervention questions either in the course chat or via the course discussion board. Students were able to post their reactions anonymously. Student responses indicated that university mental health tools are welcomed by students, but, importantly, many had not known or had forgotten about them. One student remarked, "Before this presentation I had no clue that the [this] campus offered all these resources for their students." Another wrote,

> I think that it is great the campus offers so many different forms of help for those who need it. As a student, knowing I can seek help within my campus at no cost to me is relieving because counseling is so expensive! Their presentation was great, and I think informing more students about these resources is a great idea.

Students were also asked if the resources on the campus mental health website would change someone's mind about getting help. One student responded, "I do think that the website could change someone's mind about getting help because it could make them realize that many people experience what they are going through and getting help isn't something to be ashamed of." Considering that one topic discussed by the counselors in the session was the stigma surrounding mental health diagnoses, it was heartening to hear this student's perspective. More importantly, it showed that students could see that the website was designed, in part, to mitigate stigma and to increase mental health help-seeking.

In the fall 2020 Counselor group, one of the counselors from the spring classes presented the same information. Much like the spring 2020 group, students' general opinions of the online resources were very positive. Three students highlighted the variety of resources available on the webpage, particularly noting the anonymous hotlines, call or text option, anonymous screening tools, and link for a counselor appointment. Five students were surprised and pleased that campus counseling was free, or rather, included in their tuition. Two others commented that the webpage was easy to find. Students characterized the resources as good (4 responses), great (8 responses), and helpful/useful (7 responses).

Postintervention Responses: Narrative Group

Our second intervention group, the Narrative group, was instructor-led. In both the spring of 2020 and the fall of 2021 terms, the instructor presented the campus mental health resource website to students in the focus group and also included narrative videos, from links on the site, of others' experiences with mental health challenges. Again, students responded that tools in general were helpful, but students had not had time nor inclination to explore them fully. After the presentation of campus mental health resources and narratives, students were asked if they had been previously aware of the existence of these resources. Three students from the spring responded that they knew there were campus mental health resources, but they had forgotten about them. These resources are mentioned (along with a great many other campus resources) in a required course for first-year students. Because students in the fall had been reminded about the resource throughout the semester, all indicated that they knew about the website, but, importantly, also indicated that they had never explored it.

All students described the mental health resources website as "easy to navigate" with "obvious" and "evident" links. They said, "it seems like anyone can get help." However, students noted some design concerns, such as, "it could be improved in that people who are having a hard time would probably not be motivated to follow through with some of the supports." Students suggested that these mental health resources should be better advertised and introduced to students by "an actual human." In a longer response, one student wrote:

> It would be more helpful if a professor presented this to students and connected it to insights from class. Students would rather talk to a human that they trust than a website. A lot of students would go to a professor, especially one who allows students to stay after to talk about projects, before a counselor.

Thus, this student not only judges that a person is preferable to a website but also believes that professors should take active roles in advocating for mental health help-seeking behaviors. After viewing the resources, students generally felt that their definition of mental health had not changed and that they might use these resources themselves in the future and would "always tell anyone about it that I feel may benefit from it." They thought that people who resist getting mental health supports might view the campus resource website favorably because "it allows them to make a choice" and would be helpful for new students.

Several questions were specific to the Narrative group and were based on students' perceptions of the narrative videos and text. Significantly, many students had not known of the existence of the videos until the instructor helped the students to navigate to them. We had anticipated, though, that students would find the narratives empowering, uplifting, or even inspiring once we brought them to their attention. Surprisingly, however, responses about the videos were indifferent or negative. In the focus group, one student said, "The celebrity stories weren't helpful for me. Their experiences are different than mine. They live drastically different lives." Another student agreed with the first, saying, "There is a gap between our lives." A third student suggested that the narratives would be "relatable" if the narratives came from other students. Nevertheless, students thought the general idea of using stories as an avenue to improve students' understanding of mental health issues was "helpful, but it comes down to every individual and how they react to it." Another student echoed this sentiment, saying that "it may work with some, may work better without it to some as well. People are unique, not one size fits all." A final opinion from a student was as follows, "It would be more helpful if a counselor or trusted instructor told stories vs. the videos." Also, while students in this group were not particularly responsive to the narratives of others that they did not know, when asked, students were drawn to spaces in which they could investigate "I" statements with mental health information that were included on the top of the "Half of Us" website. For example, three students commented on the ease of finding a mental health concern that they identified with and appreciated that they could, then, with a click of a button, find online mental health suggestions that correlated with the statement. All students, however, said that this feature should link to university counseling supports—particularly with a link to a local counselor vs. a national number. These responses indicate that prerecorded narratives that rely on student navigation may be less compelling than human-engaged discussions about mental health resources. Students' responses also suggest that if a website frames common mental health concerns as "I feel" statements that students can choose from and identify with, particularly when such features are accompanied by mental health definitions in lay person's terms and with "in time" strategies that correlate with the issue, students might engage more in these online spaces.

Suggestions for Implementation

Overall, we found that students were not aware of university mental health resources, yet they viewed them favorably after the intervention. Unexpectedly, though, students did not feel connected to the current narratives available on the campus mental health resource webpage. However, student feedback on the narratives indicated that the stories could be helpful if they were more relatable or if students could imagine themselves as part of the narrative. We see this feedback as particularly valuable and hope to use our results to clarify definitions about mental health and to improve students' perceptions of our campus' mental health resources.

We were surprised that students in both the Counselor and Narrative groups either did not know about our campus mental health resources or had been told once and forgotten about their existence. While students had varied responses about how their definitions of mental health concerns changed, they were not aware of university-sponsored links. Instead, students believed they would tell someone who needed mental health supports to find a local counselor or seek out a trusted adult, such as a friend or family member. In most cases, this friend or family member would not have any training in mental health issues, diagnosis, or therapy techniques. It is conceivable that this advice would, then, do more harm than good, depending on the nature of the mental health concern. While the person may receive some emotional support from a trusted adult, only a licensed counselor should be providing mental health therapy, bringing up concerns about student's perceptions of ethos, disclosure, and mental health. That students in our focus groups were unaware of our campus mental health resources is worrisome enough, but equally concerning is that they had forgotten of their existence after an introduction (usually in their freshman year). This result indicates that telling students about these resources once, particularly as part of a long list of other campus resources, is insufficient.

We also observed a preference for "choice," or a sense of agency in student responses. Students felt that seeking counseling should always be a choice; they also wanted choices in how that counseling could occur, so different ways of rhetorically framing mental health supports appealed to different audience members. The mental health resources included hotlines, but also numbers that could be texted. Many of our current students feel more comfortable texting than speaking on the phone, so the choice of talking or texting was viewed positively by students. Students liked that the resources themselves were varied, including hotlines for specific reasons (e.g., domestic violence) and groups (e.g., veterans), anonymous screenings, and direct links to set up either an in-person or phone appointment with a campus counselor. Overall, students felt that the varied options for mental health assistance were helpful and necessary.

One of the most illuminating aspects of our findings was when students pointed out parts of the websites that were not compelling and what they would do to make the sites more engaging. As part of the focus group conversation, for instance, we asked our students, in both the Counselor and Narrative focus groups, for specific changes that would improve the online resources. Students' main suggestion was to better advertise the resources to students. They suggested social media, mass text messages, on-campus postings, and targeted emails. Seven students thought it would be beneficial if these resources were discussed in multiple classes by multiple professors and also by having more professors invite counselors to class. Thus, an important intervention into mental health we suggest is that those of us working in technical communication help with user testing of and share revision ideas for online mental health tools at our home institutions. Another suggestion is that all teaching staff in higher education take an active role in promoting mental health services on their campuses.

Likewise, the advice students in our focus groups offer could be of immediate use to counseling centers as they do internal audits of their online tools. Students in our focus groups thought that the webpage could be improved by adding a video by the local counselor to introduce themselves and a video explaining how to sign up for one-on-one counseling. Ten students specifically asked for more "visible" links to sign up for counseling. In addition to a more visible counseling sign up link, they think the anonymous (i.e., confidential) nature of counseling should be better emphasized. Two students suggested a new form of communication be used—a way to email a counselor questions and get an email back. Also, three students suggested that there should be more spaces for positive information on the site, as in places that discuss proactive measures for mental wellness.

Significantly, in the Narrative group, the mental health resources website was viewed favorably, yet the narratives embedded in them were not. Students largely rejected the ethos of the subjects in the videos they viewed. Students thought the website should be better advertised in general, but that it would be much more helpful if mental health resources were introduced by professors with whom they had a relationship. In both groups, students suggested that if multiple professors presented this information throughout their college years, students would certainly be less likely to forget it. Students also suggested that the current narratives be replaced with stories featuring fellow students. The narratives could, then, be more effectively presented by a counselor (as a guest in the classroom) or by their professor.

Based on the feedback we received, we make the following additional conclusions and recommendations: (1) Students responded to human guidance through the university mental health resources: both instructor-led and counselor-led interventions are helpful to students, (2) Mental health resources need to be frequently advertised using multiple formats and in multiple contexts, (3) Narratives should be relatable to students and should consider students themselves as authorized to create their own mental health narrative through "I" statements, and (4) Links to counselors should be visible and emphasize the face-to-face format and confidentiality of sessions.

Our suggestions are in line with other works in this collection that examine university mental health interventions, yet our study does not do the important work that Leslie Angelsey and Adam Hubrig's chapter does, which is examining how mental health is presented to students as a mandate through which they might achieve academic success or might reach other metrics of traditional, neoliberal successes. Taken together, our chapters might offer a variety of specific interventions for university counseling centers looking for ways to enhance mental health help-seeking on their campuses. Likewise, our chapter works well with Lynn Reid's chapter, which outlines a training program for university instructors to help to contest stigmas and allow instructors to come from a place of rhetorical empathy in responding to students' mental health struggles.

Still, we feel that additional rhetorical research is warranted to further understand how university ethos impacts mental health help-seeking, particularly in response to students' focus group discussions of a preference for initial human interaction to introduce tools that might be paired with other preferences, such as texting features. Also, these initial responses suggest that more research about how students engage with and/or identify (or not) with definitions and narratives about mental health as represented on sites could yield important insights about how students might interact with tools and how tools might be improved.

Note

1 IRB # 20-133.

References

Angelsey, Leslie, & Hubrig, Adam. (2021). "Do you feel like :(": Discursive interventions in university mental health rhetorics. In Lisa Melonçon and Cathryn Molloy (Eds.), *Strategic interventions in mental health rhetoric.* (p. 185–205). Routledge.

Charmaz, Kathy. (2006). *Constructing grounded theory: A practical guide through qualitative analysis.* Sage.

Charon, Rita. (2001). Narrative medicine: A model for empathy, reflection, profession, and trust. *JAMA, 286*(15), 1897–1902. doi:10.1001/jama.286.15.1897

Farrer, Louise, Gulliver, Amelia, Chan, Jade Ky, Bennett, Kylie, & Griffiths, Kathleen M. (2015). A virtual mental health clinic for university students: A qualitative study of end-user needs and priorities. *JMIR Mental Health, 2*(1). doi:10.2196/mental.3890

Harrer, Mathias, Adam, Sophia, H., Baumeister, Harald, Cuijpers, Pim, Karyotaki, Eirini, Auerbach, Randy, P., Kessler, Ronald, C., Bruffaerts, Ronny, Berking, Matthias, & Ebert, David. (2018). Internet interventions for mental health in university students: A systematic review and meta-analysis. *International Journal of Methods in Psychiatric Research, 28*(2), 1–18. https://doi.org/10.1002/mpr.1759

Hartrey, Laura, Denieffe, Suzanne, & Wells, John, S.G. (2017). A systemic review of barriers and supports to the participation of students with mental health difficulties in higher education. *Mental Health & Prevention, 6,* 26–43. https://doi.org/10.1016/j.mhp.2017.03.002

Holladay, Drew. (2017). Classified conversations: Psychiatry and tactical technical communication in online spaces. *Technical Communication Quarterly, 26*(1), 8–24. doi:10.1080/10572252.2016.1257744

Lattie, Emily G., Lipson, Sarah Ketchen, & Eisenberg, Daniel. (2019). Technology and college student mental health: challenges and opportunities. *Frontiers in Psychiatry, 10,* 1–5. doi:10.3389/fpsyt.2019.00246

Melonçon, Lisa, & Frost, Erin A. (2015). Charting an emerging field: The rhetorics of health and medicine and its importance in communication design. *Communication Design Quarterly, 3*(4), 7–14.

Reid, Lynn. (2021). Toward an empathy-first approach to student mental health: A guide for faculty development. In Lisa Melonçon and Cathryn Molloy (Eds). *Strategic interventions in mental health rhetoric* (p. xx). Routledge.

Reynolds, J. Fred. (2018). A short history of mental health rhetoric research (MHRR). *Rhetoric of Health & Medicine, 1*(1–2), 1–18. doi:10.5744/rhm.2018.1003

Ryan, Megan L., Shochet, Ian, M., & Stallman, Helen, M. (2010). Universal online interventions might engage psychologically distressed university students who are unlikely to seek formal help. *Advances in Mental Health, 9*(1), 73–83. doi:10.5172/jamh.9.1.73

Scott, J. Blake, & Melonçon, Lisa. (2018). Manifesting methodologies for the rhetoric of health & medicine. In L. Melonçon & J. B. Scott (Eds.), *Methodologies for the rhetoric of health & medicine* (pp. 1–23). Routledge.

Scholten, Hanneke, & Granic, Isabela. (2019). Using the principles of design thinking to address limitations of digital mental health interventions for youth. *Journal of Medical Internet Research, 21*(2).doi:10.2196/11528

Uthappa, N. Renuka. (2017). Moving closer: Speakers with mental disabilities, deep disclosure, and agency through vulnerability. *Rhetoric Review, 36*(2), 164–175. doi:10.1080/07350198.2017.1282225

INDEX

Note: **Bold** page numbers refer to tables; page numbers followed by "n" denote endnotes.